# LASER KERATECTOMY: APPROACHES, COMPLICATIONS AND EFFECTIVENESS

# Laser Keratectomy: Approaches, Complications and Effectiveness

Luis W. Schröder
and
Felix J. Walter
Editors

**Nova Science Publishers, Inc.**
*New York*

For permission to use material from this book please contact us:
Telephone 631-231-7269; Fax 631-231-8175
Web Site: http://www.novapublishers.com



**Library of Congress Cataloging-in-Publication Data**

Laser keratectomy : approaches, complications, and effectiveness / [edited by] Luis W. Schröder and Felix J. Walter.
p. ; cm.
Includes bibliographical references and index.
ISBN 978-1-60456-863-9 (hardcover)
1. Cornea--Laser surgery. 2. Refractive keratoplasty. I. Schröder, Luis W. II. Walter, Felix J.
[DNLM: 1. Corneal Surgery, Laser. WW 340 L343 2008]
RE336.L265 2008
617.7'190598--dc22

20080262

*Published by Nova Science Publishers, Inc. ✢ New York*

# Contents

# Preface

Keratotomy is a surgical incision (a cut) made into the cornea. A radial keratotomy is a surgical procedure designed to flatten the cornea, reduce its optical power, and correct nearsightedness (myopia). The procedure is called a radial keratotomy because the incisions resemble the spokes in a bicycle wheel. The pioneer of modern laser keratectomy was the late S.N. Fyodorov in Russia.

Chapter I - Though modern refractive surgery techniques have been developed over the past 30 years, attempts to correct nearsightedness without the use of glasses have been ongoing for centuries. Ancient Chinese reportedly placed sandbags over their eyes while sleeping to flatten their corneas as an attempt to improve their vision.

The first modern push towards non-spectacle vision correction began when Frans Cornelius Donders, a Dutch physician, systematically described the anomalies of accommodation and their optical and clinical aspects in 1864. His report started the first movement to surgically correct refractive error. Several techniques were attempted, from simply removing healthy lenses to removing the vitreous, often with disastrous results, all in an attempt to change the refractive power or length of the axis of the eye. During this time, Dr. J. Ball promoted a device to "restore eyesight and render spectacles useless". This device consisted of a small, spring-loaded mallet mounted on an eye cup. It reportedly restored sight by pounding the cornea flat by striking it through a closed eyelid. Charles Tyrrell aggressively marketed his Ideal Sight Restorer, which was composed of a U-shaped device with eye cups and a rubber bulb at the base that purportedly improved vision by massaging the eyes.

A more scientific method towards developing a viable method of refractive surgery began in 1898 with Dutch physican Leendert Jan Lans. Working on his doctorate, Lans published the results of experiments on rabbits to treat astigmatism using keratectomy, keratotomy and themokeratoplasty. He found that the cornea could flatten in the perpendicular meridian when a transverse incision was made. He concluded that the incision would have to be deep to have any effect, and this effect would often be lost as the incision healed.

In 1936 Tsutomu Sato observed corneal flattening in a keratoconus patient due to spontaneous breaks in Descemet's membrane[7]. Three years later he developed a technique to cure keratoconus, astigmatism and myopia though anterior and posterior incisions of the cornea. Though the incisions worked to change the corneal curvature and improve visual acuity, the posterior incisions disrupted the endothelium. Unfortunately, the corneal endothelium's role in maintaining clarity had not been elucidated at the time, and most of his patients later developed bullos keratopathy.

Sato's pioneering work was further developed by Svyatoslov Fyodorov of the Soviet Union. Fyodorov first learned of Sato's research and surgical techniques while attending the Japanese Ophthalmologic Conference in Niigata, Japan in 1960. It wasn't until 1972, when Fyodorov treated a 16 year old patient with corneal lacerations from shattered glasses, that he made a breakthrough in keratotomy. He found that precise, radial cuts at the anterior cornea, determined by a mathematical formula he devised to adjust to various corneal curvatures, provided him the ability to control the amount of visual correction.

Radial keratotomy was the first refractive procedure to gain widespread acceptance among the medical field. In the meantime, the excimer laser was being developed as a precursor to today's modern refractive surgical techniques.

Chapter II - Different corneal refractive procedures are used to correct ametropias. In the 1950's, Barraquer described the first corneal procedures with corneal keratomileusis to correct low, moderate and high myopia and hyperopia. In the 1970's, Fyodorov and Durnev described radial keratectomy to correct myopia. In the 1980's, Trokel described the use of the excimer laser in refractive corneal surgery with Photorefractive Keratectomy (PRK), and at the end of the decade McDonald and Pallikaris described Laser-Assisted in Situ Keratomileusis (LASIK). Today, laser procedures are the most frequent corneal refractive surgeries, with techniques such as Photorefractive Keratectomy (PRK), Laser-Assisted in-situ Keratomileusis (LASIK) and Wavefront-guided LASIK, and Conductive keratoplasty (CK).

Photorefractive Keratectomy (PRK) applies excimer laser ablation directly to the Bowman membrane after corneal des-epithelisation. This technique is safe and effective for correcting low ametropias (lower than 6.00 D).

Laser-Assisted in-situ Keratomileusis (LASIK) applies excimer laser ablation to the stroma after making a corneal flap. It is safe and effective for correcting low and moderate myopia and low hyperopia with or without moderate astigmatism. Different software makes it possible to correct optical aberrations of the eye, such as coma, spherical aberration and others, with wave-front guided LASIK.

More recently, Conductive Keratoplasty (CK) using a holmium laser has been approved by the FDA to correct low hyperopia and presbyopia. This procedure applies a holmium laser to the corneal periphery to steepen the corneal curvature.

Chapter III – Introduction: Infections are potentially devastating in ocular surgery and several reviews and multicenter trials have been dealing with infection following cataract surgery. Both in LASIK and in PRK infections might have a serious course and determine poor refractive results and in some cases lead to keratoplasty.

Matherial and methods: a meta-analysis of the literature was performed. PRK and LASIK were considered separately.

Results: Infections following refractive surgery (both PRK and LASIK) are extremely rare. The great majority of infections were caused by gram positive bacteria. Preferred therapy is by fourth generation fluoroquinolones. There is no accepted prevention of the infection in the literature. When comparing the occurrence of infections in PRK and LASIK similar prevalence was found.

Conclusions: Although rare, infections following refractive surgery are potentially devastating. Accurate prevention of infection is described in this review. Most of the infections occur during the first week and accurate follow up is recommended during the first few days following the procedure. Identification of the infective agent is important in order to start a targeted therapy.

Chapter IV- The alcohol-assisted manual technique used to lift the corneal epithelium during laser-assisted subepithelial keratectomy (LASEK) often results in stretching of the epithelial flap, causing the flap edges to overlap the border of peripheral epithelium. We describe a lift-and-scrape technique that entails the creation of a smaller flap and the subsequent removal of enough peripheral epithelium to allow for flap stretching. This avoids potential problems associated with epithelial overlap while at the same time improving the ease of flap creation.

Chapter V - The risk of postoperative flap dislocation, iatrogenic ectasia, epithelial ingrowth and other complications of laser in situ keratomileusis (LASIK) have led to renewed interest in surface ablation techniques. Photorefractive keratectomy (PRK) performed with and without the use of mitomycin-C (MMC), laser epithelial keratomileusis (LASEK) and epithelial laser in situ keratomileusis (Epi-LASIK) are all used extensively in the U.S. military. Research into the long term outcomes of surface ablation techniques is currently underway at Walter Reed Army Medical Center. In this paper we review the scientific rationale, indications, techniques, and outcomes for advanced surface ablations at Walter Reed Army Medical Center.

Chapter VI – The first goal of a laser treatment for refractive surgery is to balance the refractive defects of an eye. The optical quality of an eye is significantly determined through low and high order aberrations. These always define an optical error, regardless of whether they are corneal or ocular aberrations.

We have low order aberrations as sphere and cylinder and high order aberrations such coma, spherical aberration, trefoil or pentafoil. It can occur, and actually, it is often the case, that the best approach for planning and ablation is a sophisticated pattern, which can still be described simply in terms of sphere, cylinder, and orientation (axis). Studies of untreated eyes show that patients with above-average visual acuity (somehow individuals achieving supervision) can have moderate amounts of high-order aberrations. It was also observed that the individuals with the least amount of aberrations were not necessarily the ones scoring the highest visual acuities. In these studies, performed among populations with supernormal vision, no direct relationship between these high-order aberrations and visual performance of untreated eyes could be determined. Moreover, because the brain adjusts to aberrations through the help of neural compensation, and these aberrations are in the experience of the patient as normal, it is not always advantageous to remove all aberrations through laser correction. There is some plasticity of the neural system so that distortions in the visual field are corrected, but as patients are viewing the world through their own wave aberration they will reject corrections which are too large from their "normal" experience. With aberration-free patterns we tailor the eye's subjective sphero-cylindrical refractive error, different of the term wavefront guided where the high order aberrations are also corrected.

Some studies on treated eyes found that wavefront guided treatments induce less aberration than conventional profiles, but they are not actually reducing the preoperative aberrations, indeed they created new ones.

In this context an „Aberration-Free" treatment is optimum for patients whose sight is not affected by existing high-order aberrations and for those who – only corrected with glasses - possess a visual acuity of 1.0 or better. With this treatment, the (pre-operative) high-order aberrations remain unchanged. The advantage is that the patient retains the habitual sight impression ("visual print") at best focus and the brain requires no learning phase to deal with otherwise added bothersome changes. The ideal profile "Aberration-Free" means that the laser treatment, with a highly sophisticated pattern is delivered in such way that only spherical and/or cylindrical refractive values are corrected. No optical high-order aberrations are changed nor additional aberrations induced that could reduce vision sharpness and contrast, as opposed to classical, Munnerlyn-based treatments and a number of aspheric methods used in the market that induce aberrations.. Thus, the pre-operative and post-operative high order aberrations are identical. So that we are treating the eye in a neutral way. The goal is to correct the manifest refraction without inducing or changing the aberrations of the eye.

If the diagnostically assessed high-order aberrations impair the visual performance, they should be corrected. In those cases we recommend wavefront-guided treatments as the right choice, when corneal and/or ocular wavefront data can be included. We should plan the most optimum ablation pattern specifically for each individual eye based on its anamnesis, diagnosis, and visual demands and allow even more individual, patient-oriented treatment.

Chapter VII - Amblyopia is one of the most common preventable causes of visual acuity loss in children.The Amblyopia Treatment Studies (ATS) report excellent results in reversing amblyopia with glasses in combination with patching, atropine treatment, or both. Conversely, the ATS studies also show that a significant subset of amblyopic patients, even without coexisting medical or ocular problems, do not have successful, timely resolution of their amblyopia with standard treatment regimens. Recently refractive surgery has been proposed in addition to standard antiamblyopic treatments, especially in patients with high refractive errors and non compliant with contact lens use.

Chapter VIII - During the last decade, advances in the knowledge and measurement of the eye's optical aberrations have moved the wave aberration theory from an obscure scientific concept to one that is central to efforts to improve vision. Nowadays, all the imperfections in the components and materials within the eye that cause light rays to deviate from the desired path are referred to as optical aberrations. Refractive surgery aims to minimize optical aberrations in the eye. Excimer laser surgery is the most performed surgical technique to improve unaided vision. The personalized correction of the eye's aberrations promises to be the next golden standard in laser refractive surgery. The technique necessitates an accurate determination of the wavefront error and a precise system of surgical correction. To date, although it has been demonstrated that image quality after customized procedures is improved over that of standard procedures, there are still significant aberrations induced after a wavefront-guided procedure that are neither expected nor predicted. The ability to anticipate confounding biophysical responses of the cornea at the level of the individual patient remains still limited and should be improved.

The development of innovative wavefront sensing and correcting methods and techniques is now opening new perspectives of high-precision refractive corrections. Data coming from the reliable measurements of the corneal and ocular wave aberration may be used to drive a more precise personalized correction of the eye's aberrations for eliminating low-order aberrations and further compensating high-order aberrations between cornea and lens to optimize the individual visual performance. Accordingly, identifying all the components of corneal biophysical response to develop therapeutic models for compensating for these factors will ultimately lead to increased predictability of visual outcomes.

Major advances in presbyopia correction are also expected in the near future, thanks to the application of innovative electro-optical technologies, such as liquid crystals, in vision science.

Short Communication A - Although the excimer laser correction of myopic and hyperopic defects has gained high levels of predictability and stability, the surface correction of presbyopia is still a matter of debate. It is well known that during accommodation in the pre-presbyopic age there is a change from slightly negative or neutral to a positive spherical aberration. Furthermore, when a hyperopic correction in a presbyopic patient is performed), it is commonly seen a better performance in near vision and a positive spherical aberration is usually induced. This observations lead to the idea that there might be a connection between spherical aberration (z4,0) and near vision. We present the 2 year's follow-up visual results of the treatment of myopic and hyperopic patients with the Zeiss Mel 70 Mel 80 excimer laser inducing a positive spherical aberration in 53 patients (Bartoli-Zeiss method).

Short Communication B - Excimer laser corneal surgery allows the precise removal of tissue and it is nowadays used worldwide for the correction of the eye's optical aberrations. During the last years, novel methods and techniques have been developed in order to improve the accuracy of surface ablation surgery. On the other hand, even in an era of high-precision treatment algorithms, discrepancies between the intended and realized visual outcomes are sometimes manifest. The biophysical responses of the cornea undermine the predictability and stability of refractive surgery and contribute to these discrepancies.

Numerous factors depending on the ablation parameters may vary the remodeling of the ablated corneal surface leading to abnormal wound healing. A smooth postoperative stromal surface is required to achieve a high-quality visual outcome. In this work, we provide nanometer-resolved images of either native or photoablated corneas to demonstrate the opportunity in which Atomic Force Microscopy (AFM) may be valuable to understand the laser-tissue interaction and characterize the three-dimensional ultra-structural changes of the corneal stroma induced by excimer laser surgery.

The stromal surface of eight porcine corneas, both natural and photoablated, was imaged with AFM operating in balanced salt solution and contact mode. The AFM images of the intact corneal stroma, exposed after chemical removal of the epithelium, showed a smooth surface with pores of varying diameter and dimension consisting in the Bowman's layer. Following ablation, the stromal surface showed undulations and micro-granular structures. These structures are considered to be either collapsed collagen fibrils and debris, directly due to the effects of laser beam impact onto the stromal surface. Topographical data, calculated using the section analysis module of the AFM software, showed an increased roughness of the post-ablated stromal surface compared to its native state, with a mean root mean square roughness value of 215 ± 49 nanometer (nm) and 144 ± 41 nm respectively. Nevertheless, the quantitative analysis proved that the laser cut of commercial excimer laser systems is very precise in removing even infinitesimally small amounts of tissue.

# Research and Review Studies

In: Laser Keratectomy: Approaches, Complications... ISBN 978-1-60456-863-9
Author: Luis W. Schröder and Felix J. Walter 

*Chapter I*

# History of Refractive Surgery

***Jayson D. Edwards and Kraig S. Bower***
Center for Refractive Surgery
Walter Reed Army Medical Center
Washington, DC, USA

## Introduction

Though modern refractive surgery techniques have been developed over the past 30 years, attempts to correct nearsightedness without the use of glasses have been ongoing for centuries. Ancient Chinese reportedly placed sandbags over their eyes while sleeping to flatten their corneas as an attempt to improve their vision [1]

The first modern push towards non-spectacle vision correction began when Frans Cornelius Donders, a Dutch physician, systematically described the anomalies of accommodation and their optical and clinical aspects in 1864[2]. His report started the first movement to surgically correct refractive error. Several techniques were attempted, from simply removing healthy lenses to removing the vitreous, often with disastrous results, all in an attempt to change the refractive power or length of the axis of the eye. During this time, Dr. J. Ball promoted a device to "restore eyesight and render spectacles useless"[3]. This device consisted of a small, spring-loaded mallet mounted on an eye cup. It reportedly restored sight by pounding the cornea flat by striking it through a closed eyelid. Charles Tyrrell aggressively marketed his Ideal Sight Restorer, which was composed of a U-shaped device with eye cups and a rubber bulb at the base that purportedly improved vision by massaging the eyes[4].

A more scientific method towards developing a viable method of refractive surgery began in 1898 with Dutch physican Leendert Jan Lans[5]. Working on his doctorate, Lans published the results of experiments on rabbits to treat astigmatism using keratectomy, keratotomy and themokeratoplasty[6]. He found that the cornea could flatten in the perpendicular meridian when a transverse incision was made. He concluded that the incision would have to be deep to have any effect, and this effect would often be lost as the incision healed.

In 1936 Tsutomu Sato observed corneal flattening in a keratoconus patient due to spontaneous breaks in Descemet's membrane[7]. Three years later he developed a technique to cure keratoconus, astigmatism and myopia though anterior and posterior incisions of the cornea[8]. Though the incisions worked to change the corneal curvature and improve visual acuity, the posterior incisions disrupted the endothelium. Unfortunately, the corneal endothelium's role in maintaining clarity had not been elucidated at the time, and most of his patients later developed bullos keratopathy[9].

Sato's pioneering work was further developed by Svyatoslov Fyodorov of the Soviet Union. Fyodorov first learned of Sato's research and surgical techniques while attending the Japanese Ophthalmologic Conference in Niigata, Japan in 1960. It wasn't until 1972, when Fyodorov treated a 16 year old patient with corneal lacerations from shattered glasses, that he made a breakthrough in keratotomy. He found that precise, radial cuts at the anterior cornea, determined by a mathematical formula he devised to adjust to various corneal curvatures, provided him the ability to control the amount of visual correction[10].

Radial keratotomy was the first refractive procedure to gain widespread acceptance among the medical field. In the meantime, the excimer laser was being developed as a precursor to today's modern refractive surgical techniques.

## The Excimer Laser

The first use of a laser in refractive surgery was done by Beckman and associates in 1980 using a carbon dioxide laser. However, corneal changes were transient and other lasers and techniques were examined. The eximer laser, originally developed in 1975[11,12], was found to be superior due to its ability to provide high energy to tissue without excessive thermal damage. John Taboada was the first to use the eximer laser on corneal tissue in 1981[13], with Trokel[14] and associates reporting in 1983 that the laser was able to ablate anterior corneal tissue predictably without damage to surrounding structures. The 193-nm argon-fluorine eximer laser, as shown by Kruger et al.[15,16], produced a smoother, more precise ablation compared to longer wavelength lasers under development.

Excimer, derived from "excited" and "dimer", describes the energy source of the laser, in which electrical energy excites argon-flourine atoms, which emit photons of light. The excimer laser operates under the concept of photoablation, in that the UV energy of the laser exceeds that of molecular covelent bonds, initiating a photochemical process[17]. Under this energy insult, the breaking chemical bonds cause an increase in pressure and eject the molecular fragments[18,19]. Higher wavelengths were found to work through a photothermal process, causing increased damage to surrounding tissue. The short 193-nm wavelength, with low repetition pulses, is able to remove tissue with very little local thermal damage [20]. The amount of tissue removed is proportional to the amount of energy that is delivered to the cornea.

Two types of delivery systems are available for the excimer laser: broad-beam and small spot scanning lasers. The broad beam approach – also known as variable-beam fixed spot

(VFS) – employs a diaphragm delivery system that acts similarly to a camera to change the aperture. This can be done by use of an iris diaphragm or variable aperture system. This method of delivery has the advantage of fast treatment times, lessening fixation loss, corneal dehydration and patient discomfort. However, the diaphragm approach also results in "step-like" ablation patterns, which is believed to result in a more aggressive healing response [21]

Small spot scanning delivery can be subdivided into flying spot and rectangular beam scanning. The beams created are small (0.2 to 1 mm), allowing versatility in patterns to alter the topography of the cornea over large treatment zones. The small beam is more homogenous and allows for overlapping and multidirectional scanning, which results in a smoother ablation profile [22,23]. The flying spot technique can be customized to achieve virtually any ablation pattern by computer controlled "pixel-by-pixel" corneal ablations[21]. This variability also allows treatment of hyperopia, asymmetrical astigmatism, and phototheraputic keratectomy (PTK). Another advantage of scanning delivery systems is that an area of the cornea is not exposed to the laser continuously, so the temperature of the corneal tissue is lower than in broad-beam lasers. The small spot delivered allows for a smaller energy source and fewer optics, though the small amount of cornea ablated also results in longer treatment times. Corneal dehydration can occur, which increases the possibility of an uneven ablation [24]. Also, patient drift tends to increase due to longer treatment times. Active eye tracking systems are used to compensate for this drift.

## Photorefractive Keratectomy

The first refractive surgery technique to make use of the excimer laser system was photorefractive keratectomy (PRK) for treatment of myopia. Seiler of Germany was the first ophthalmologist to use the excimer laser for PRK ablations on humans [25]. The eyes used were blind or were to be enucleated. He followed this up later in 1987 with the first PRK ablation on a well-functioning eye [26]. L'Esperance was the first to perform PRK in the United States[27], and today the procedure is still considered an excellent technique with few serious complications. Though currently not as popular as laser in situ keratomileusis (LASIK), PRK is advantageous in its reliable safety and predictability in low to moderate myopes. Higher myopic correction is limited by increased corneal haze, pain and myopic regression[28,29,30,31].

## Indications for PRK

The decision to undergo refractive surgery rests with the patient, as does the choice of which procedure to receive. LASIK is the most common refractive surgery today, though the number of PRK procedures is increasing. Many patients are now opting for surface ablation procedures over LASIK due to excellent visual outcomes and a better safety profile. LASIK complications that are of concern include postsurgical traumatic flap dislocations, free caps, incomplete or irregular flaps, flap wrinkles or striae, buttonholes, flap melts, diffuse lamellar keratitis, corneal ectasia, epithelial defects, epithelial ingrowth and microbial keratitis[32,33,34,35,36,37,38,39,40,41]. PRK, however, is not without its complications, many of which LASIK is able to overcome. PRK complications include subepithelial haze, a lengthened recovery time and postoperative discomfort.

PRK is preferred in patients that have a history of recurrent erosions or anterior basement membrane dystrophies, as LASIK can exacerbate these conditions[42]. Lee and associates found that patients receiving PRK had a decreased incidence of postsurgical dry eye than in patients that underwent LASIK[43]. Patients that have low myopia, and as such low risk of haze formation may also do better with PRK. Additionally, PRK can be used in patients that have had previous surgery, such as radial keratectomy or LASIK[44].

In LASIK a hinged flap 80 to 200 μm is created using a microkeratome. In order to create this flap a suction ring is used on the eye, which temporarily results in an intraocular pressure (IOP) that can be greater than 65 mm Hg. PRK is recommended for glaucoma patients as the increased pressure of the suction ring in LASIK is contraindicated. In addition, patients that have deep orbits, poor exposure or anteriorly placed scleral buckles are more likely to have complications induced during flap creation. Patients with thin corneas in which the residual bed thickness under a LASIK flap is less than 250-300 μm, flat corneas (40 diopters or less) or very steep corneas (48 to 50 diopters) are best managed with PRK. In addition, patients at risk of corneal ectasia from forme fruste keratoconus or asymmetric astigmatism are also better PRK candidates[45].

Lifestyle must also be considered, as patients that are active in contact sports or in the military are at risk for postoperative flap dislocation after LASIK. Finally, a surgeon's experience should also be taken into account, as those that perform refractive surgery infrequently may be better with the less complicated PRK procedure[46].

## Surgical Technique

The goal of PRK is to change of the change the shape of the cornea, thus eliciting a change in its refractive power. This is accomplished in a two-step process – removal of the epithelium and laser treatment of the stroma.

Epithelial removal can be accomplished several different ways – mechanical, chemical or laser removal. Mechanical removal entails using a surgical blade or a rotating brush. Using a blade or spatula has been employed since the early days of surface ablation. Scraping the epithelium with a blade is carefully done, starting with the periphery to protect the central corneal and prevent dehydration. However, it may leave an irregular border or nicks in Bowman's layer. Alternatively, an Amoils or Pallikaris brush may be used to brush away the epithelium. Epithelial debris are wiped from the exposed stroma with a moistened sponge or spatula.

The basis of chemical removal of the epithelium is to disrupt the demosomes and hemidesmosomes that anchor the epithelial cells together. Several chemicals have been used to achieve this, including proparacaine, tetracaine, iodine, cocaine, lidocaine and n-heptanol. Topical anesthetics were effective, but took several minutes to work. Today 18-20% ethanol, which takes only 15 to 20 seconds, is the most commonly used chemical for epithelial debridement. In this technique the ethanol is either placed in a well or soaked in a sponge which is positioned on the cornea. This rapidly loosens the epithelium, which can then be scraped away. However, alcohol can be toxic to the epithelium and stroma as well as dehydrate the cornea.

Removal of the epithelium can also be done by the excimer laser in a process called transepithelial ablation. The central epithelium is approximately 50 μm thick and can be ablated under cobalt blue fluorescence. When the epithelium is removed and Bowman's layer exposed the fluorescence dissipates. However, the endpoint of epithelial removal is difficult to determine visually and there is variability of thickness of the epithelium over the cornea, which may lead to over or under ablation. Many practitioners have adopted laser scrape it its stead, in which the epithelium is deliberately ablated to a thickness of 40 μm, and the remaining basal layer is removed by mechanical debridement.

Since the first PRK procedure, laser technology and software have evolved and improved. The size of the ablation zone has also increased. To minimize the depth of ablation, the ablation zone initially was 3.5 to 4 mm. However, that caused edge glare and light sensitivity, especially at night. The ablation zone now is designed to be larger than the patient's fully dilated pupil, usually 5 to 8 mm, with smoothing of the edge at the transition zone. Ablation is then done in this area in a multizone/multipass technique in order to decrease corneal heating and provide a smoother ablation contour. Central corneal ablations are done in myopic patients, and peripheral ablations in hyperopic patients. A cross-cylinder ablation has been successful in patients with astigmatism.

Postoperatively, patients received a bandage contact lens that protects the de-epithelialized cornea. Lenses are generally worn for 4 to 5 days to reduce pain and aid the healing process. High oxygen permeable contact lenses are gaining greater use as they have been shown to result in faster corneal re-epithelialization and decreased pain (unpublished results). The postoperative epithelial defect increases susceptibility to bacterial keratitis, so topical antibiotics are provided. These are generally fluoroquinolones, which have broad spectrum coverage and excellent ocular tolerance[47]. Topical steroids are also provided to patients as the damaged stromal cells release cytokines, decreasing the incidence of sterile infiltrates and subepithelial haze.

## Complications of Wound Healing and Current Treatments

Though intraoperative and postoperative complications associated with PRK are uncommon, the increased incidence in corneal haze is of particular concern, especially in patients with higher degrees of myopia (greater than -6.00 diopters). Early haze formation is generally associated with wound healing, while late onset haze has been found to have a strong correlation to increased sensitivity to ultraviolet light following PRK. In addition, post-surgical regression is thought to be influenced by wound healing.

Epithelial wound healing occurs immediately after refractive surgery, controlled by cytokine mediators produced from stromal keratocytes and fibroblasts as well as lacrimal growth factors, such as tear fluid transforming growth factor-β1 (TGF- β1)[48,49]. Normally protected by the overlying epithelium, the corneal stroma responds to these lacrimal-gland derived growth factors, causing the activation and proliferation of keratocytes and resultant differentiation of fibroblasts and myofibroblasts. Each of these cell types participates in corneal haze. Preoperative keratocytes have a very low reflectivity of light. Following laser ablation, the keratocytes in the ablation zone become activated and highly reflective[50]. Fibroblasts and myofibroblasts also contribute to corneal haze due to their opacity[51]. In addition, the collagen produced by myofibroblasts is highly disorganized, lacking the ordered structure needed for transparency[52,53]. Patients with higher myopic correction require deeper ablation, resulting in a larger number of activated keratocytes, and a strong correlation between the degree of myopia and the degree of haze formation[54,55].

Epithelial hyperplasia has been shown to occur in both PRK[56] and LASIK[57], resulting in myopic regression. It is believed that this hyperplasia is associated with high levels of cytokines produced from corneal keratocytes, fibroblasts and myofibroblasts. Hepatocyte growth factor (HGF) and keratinocyte growth factor (KGF) are thought to be these modulators of epithelial proliferation[58]. This epithelial hyperplasia can be permanent.

Topical corticosteroids are often used postoperatively to treat both haze and regression. It is not clear, however, if steroids actually decrease the incidence of haze, and prolonged used can lead to adverse effects such as increases in intraocular pressure, band keratopathy and cataracts. Some studies have shown no benefit from steroids, others have shown a transient effect on haze that lasts only until steroids are discontinued[59,60,61].

The use of Mitomycin-C (0.02%) has been advanced as a solution in prevention and treatment of corneal haze by inhibiting the activation of keratocytes, resulting in decreased formation of haze. Phototheraputic keratectomy (PTK) or corneal scraping are used as treatments for haze formation, though the haze often recurs. Using mitomycin-C as an adjunct to these treatments has been effective in preventing haze from returning. In a study by Vigo et al. 100% of eyes that had developed moderate to severe haze following PRK showed improvement, up to 6 lines, in best corrected visual acuity following scraping and treatment with 0.02% mitomycin-C for 2 minutes[62]. Raviv et al. reported improvement in best corrected and uncorrected visual acuity in all 30 eyes treated with mitomycin-C after post-PRK haze formation[63]. In addition to treatment, mitomycin-C has also been shown to prevent haze formation. In a study of 60 eyes treated with PRK, 30 eyes were immediately treated with mitomycin-C. None of the 30 eyes treated with mitomycin-C developed more than trace haze, while 19 of the control eyes developed mild to severe haze[64].

Additional treatments of corneal haze include oral ascorbic acid prophylaxis and topical thiotepa. Ascorbic acid has been found to diminish an excessive wound response by decreasing keratocyte activation and protecting against UV damage[65,66]. Thiotepa, an antineoplastic agent, has been shown to successfully reduce haze in patients who didn't respond to conventional treatment[67].

## Laser Subepithelial Keratomileusis

Though LASIK is by far the most popular photorefractive technique used today, surface ablation techniques have again gained interest as surgeons endeavor to overcome the complications of creating a corneal flap. Laser subepithelial keratomileusis (LASEK), first described by Massimo Camellin[68] in 1999, is a modification of PRK in which dilute ethanol is used to loosen the epithelial adhesions from the underlying Bowman's layer. In contrast to PRK, the epithelium is repositioned following laser ablation.

## Indications

LASEK, in theory, incorporates the most beneficial aspects of both PRK and LASIK. As it is a surface ablation procedure, its safety and predictability profile are similar to PRK. There is no intrastromal incision so the technique does not suffer from flap complications seen in LASIK. The repositioned epithelial flap decreases both the amount of postoperative pain and the potential for the development of corneal haze by cytokine mediators, two significant drawbacks to PRK[69]

The most ideal candidates are those with mild to moderate myopia up to -7.00 diopters, thin corneas, anterior basement membrane disease, individuals involved in contact sports or the military, and other indications similar to PRK. However, LASEK incorporates the advantages of LASIK, including reduced postoperative pain and corneal opacities, rapid visual recovery and faster stabilization of refractive regression. The differences between LASEK, PRK and LASIK are only observed in the first few weeks, with long term visual outcome similar in all three techniques.

## Surgical Technique

There are several different techniques that can be used in LASEK, all derived from the used of chemical epithelial removal seen in PRK. The first technique used was the Camellin technique[68], which begins with a pre-cut epithelial trephination that allows greater access of the ethanol to the basement membrane. The trephine has a 90 degree blunt area at the 12 o'clock position for the hinge. A holding well is placed on the cornea and filled with 18 to 20% ethanol solution for 25 to 30 seconds. The cornea is rinsed and a spatula used to reflect the epithelial flap.

The Azar technique begins with labeling the cornea with overlapping 3 mm circles for positioning[70]. A semi-sharp well is place on the cornea and filled with ethanol, after which a modified Vannas scissors is used peripherally to cut the flap. The epithelial flap can then be peel back using a Merocel sponge.

Vinciguerra developed his technique in order to preserve epithelial attachment to the limbal stem cells[71]. Called the butterfly technique, a paracentral cut is made instead of a peripheral cut. This cut allows the formation of two flaps, which can then be reflected back to expose the stroma.

McDonald's technique[72] the does not require the use of ethanol and is loosely based off the butterfly technique. After trephination, a cataract blade is used to score the epithelium peripherally down to Bowman's layer. Viscous gel can then be injected under the epithelium, elavating the flap. A paracentral cut is then made with Vannas scissors and the two flaps resected back.

The purpose of any of these techniques is to expose the corneal stroma for laser ablation. The epithelial flap, retained with a hinge, can then be placed back into position and a bandage contact lens fit upon completion.

## Ethanol Toxicity

The major detrimental factor of LASEK procedures stems from the toxicity of ethanol to the corneal epithelium. Cell viability is determined by ethanol concentration and exposure time. Previous studies have determined that a concentration of 20% ethanol placed on the cornea for 20 seconds causes death in about 20% of cells. After 30 seconds of exposure 30% of the cells were dead and after 40 seconds 90% were dead[73]. Though the current protocol allows for 80% of the cells to be retained, there is still concern for the overall viability of the epithelial flap. Whether the flap readheres to the stroma, or simply acts as biological bandage until new epithelium grows in its stead is still a subject of debate.

## Epithelial Laser in Situ Keratomileusis (EPI-LASIK)

Epi-LASIK, a variation of LASEK, has recently emerged in an effort to combat the risk of ethanol toxicity to the corneal epithelium and stroma. First described by Ioannis Pallikaris[74], this technique incorporates the use of a microkeratome-like device that mechanically separates the epithelial cells from Bowman's layer.

## Indications

Patient selection for those receiving Epi-LASIK is similar to other surface ablation profiles. Proponents of this technique state that healing times and haze formations are decreased compared to PRK. Candidates are those with low to moderate myopia, thinner corneal thickness, steep or flat corneas or other contraindications of LASIK. Ethanol is not used for the creation of the epithelial flap and has no inherent risk or complication of ethanol toxicity seen in LASEK. Additionally, some patients may express anxiety towards a corneal stromal cut of LASIK, and the bladeless technique of Epi-LASIK can be an alternative.

## Surgical Technique

Mechanical exposure of the stroma is the defining feature of Epi-LASIK. A modified microkeratome is used to create the epithelial flap. This epimicrokeratome uses a suction ring and a blunt oscillating seperator to detach the epithelium, leaving a 2 to 3 mm nasal hinge. The epithelial flap can then be reflected back and laser ablation done on the stroma. A bandage contact lens is placed postoperatively. Designed to eliminate the complications of ethanol exposure, the Epi-LASIK microkeratome is supposed to preserve the basement membrane by placing the cleavage plane beneath it. However, due to variability of eyes, the cleavage plane has been inconsistent with reports of microfocal damage to the lamina densa[75].

## Surface Ablations at Walter Reed Army Medical Center

Though LASIK is the most popular method in most corneal refractive surgery practices, most military personnel do not qualify for LASIK due to the risk of traumatic postoperative flap dislocation, and in general undergo surface ablation procedures. PRK is the most common surface ablation techniques used in the military[76]. However, concerns over post-PRK haze have lead refractive surgeons to find alternative surface ablation techniques. Several small case series, clinical trials and anecdotal experiences suggest that there is a lower incidence of haze associated with mitomycin C PRK (MMC PRK) and LASEK than there is with PRK. An ongoing prospective clinical study at the Walter Reed Army Medical Center's Center for Refractive Surgery is underway to determine differences in visual outcomes among the three procedures and to help standardize care.

## Patients and Methods

A total of 167 patients (334 eyes) underwent surface ablation treatment. Patients were randomized to treatment of their dominant eye with either MMC PRK (0.1 mg/ml x 1 minute) or LASEK. The fellow eye received conventional PRK. Inclusion criteria included age 21 or above, manifest refractive spherical equivalent between -4.00 diopters and -10.00 diopters, refractive stability and best spectacle corrected visual acuity (BACVA) of 20/20 or better in both eyes. Exclusion criteria included female subjects who are pregnant who intend to become pregnant, residual, recurrent or active ocular disease, any medical condition that may impair healing, such as collagen vascular disease, autoimmune disease, ocular herpes infections or immunodeficiency disease, and current use of topical or systemic medications that impair healing, including corticosteroids, antimetabolites, etc.

All individuals received surface ablation using LADARVision$^{TM}$ excimer laser system (Alcon Surgical, Ft. Worth, Texas). Patients received topical tetracoine 0.5% prior to treatment. Eyes undergoing PRK (n = 167) or MMC PRK (n = 85) had the corneal epithelium removed with the used of an Amoils rotary brush. Eyes that underwent LASEK had a 9.0 mm flap created by use of a trephine, in which the hinge was positioned superiorly. The epithelial flap was loosened using 20% ethanol for 25 to 35 seconds and reflected superiorly using a spatula. After surface ablation, eyes receiving MMC PRK had a cornea light shield soaked with 0.02% mitomycin-C placed on the ablation zone and left in place for 60 seconds, after which the cornea was irrigated with one 30 ml bottle of chilled BSS. All eyes received postoperative moxifloxacin 0.5% and ketoralc 0.5% with placement of a bandage soft contact lens.

Patients returned for postoperative care at 1 day, 4 days and 1 week, with follow up examinations at 1, 3, 6 and 12 months. Visual outcomes measurements were taken at follow up visits, including uncorrected visual acuity (UCVA), best spectacle corrected visual acuity (BSCVA), manifest refraction, and 5% and 25% low contrast visual acuity (LCVA). Endothelial cell counts were assessed at 6 ant 12 months. UCVA and BSCVA measurements were taken using a 4 meter LogMAR back-illuminated eye chart (Lighthouse Second edition, New York, NY). A standardized phoropter with a vertex distance of 12.5 mm was used to evaluate manifest refraction. LCVA was assessed with the Precision Vision Optical series of LogMAR charts with back illumination at 5% and 25% contrast. Haze rate was recorded on a scale of 0 to 4. Endothelial cell counts were assessed with the ConfoScan4 confocal microscope (Nidek Technologies, Albignasego, Italy).

Results were recorded using an Excel spreadsheet (Microsoft Corp, Redmont, Washington), and data were analyzed using SPSS for Windows version 15.0 (SPSS Inc., Chicago, Illinois) using Mann-Whitney tests. A P values of <0.5 was considered statistically significant.

## Results

A total of 167 eyes underwent PRK, 84 eyes underwent MMC PRK and 83 eyes underwent LASEK. The mean patient age was 35 (range 21 to 57), with 57 female and 110 male patients. The preoperative mean spherical equivalent was -5.61 ±1.44 D (range 2.75 to -9.25 D), mean cylinder was -0.78 ±0.69 D (range 0 to -3.25 D) and mean manifest spherical equivalent was -6.00 ±1.42 D (range -3.88 to -9.38 D).

## Safety

The number of eyes losing two or more lines of BSCVA was used as a measurement of safety. At one month 4.3% of PRK, 4.8% of MMC PRK and 2.4% of LASEK eyes lost two or more lines BSCVA. At 3 months 1 PRK eye and 1 MMC PRK eye continued to have 2 or more lines lost of BSCVA. One patient that received PRK in one eye and LASEK in the other lost 3 lines bilaterally at 6 months due to 2+ corneal haze. One additional PRK eye lost 3 lines BSCVA at the 12 month post-op visit due to 2+ late onset corneal haze. The patient's alternate eye underwent LASEK and gained one line of BSCVA. This patient had no previous complications prior to 12 months. Both patients with late onset haze were treated with corneal scraping and MMC, with resolution of the haze and improvement in visual acuity to 20/20 or better.

# Efficacy

Efficacy was measured by UCVA of 20/20 and 20/40 and better. Results are shown in Figure 1. At one month more LASEK eyes (64.6%) compared to MMC PRK eyes (43.3%) had a postoperative visual acuity of 20/20 ($p=0.006$). Differences between groups were insignificant after 1 month.

Comparing pre-operative BSCVA with post-operative UCVA also provides a valuable test to evaluate efficacy. At one month postoperatively, UCVA was within one line of the pre-op BSCVA in 66.2% of LASEK eyes compared to 51.8% of MMC PRK eyes ($p = 0.12$). There was no significant difference between groups after the first post-operative month (Figure 2).

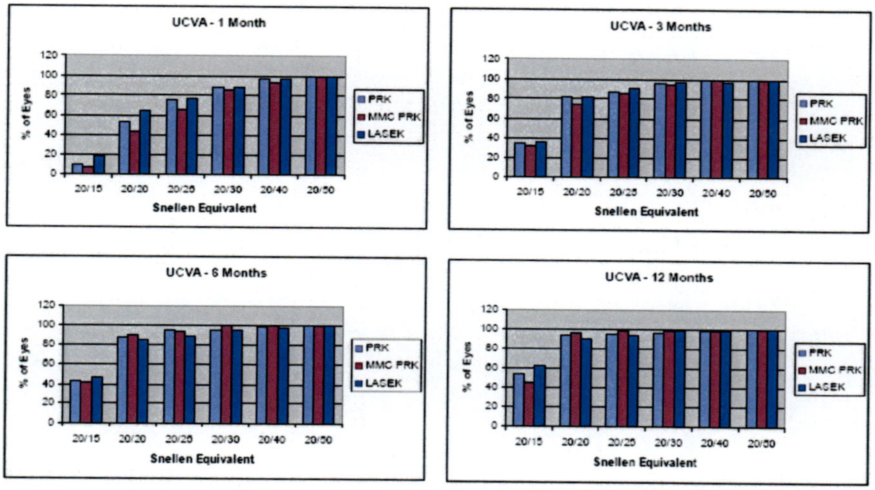


Figure 1. UCVA.

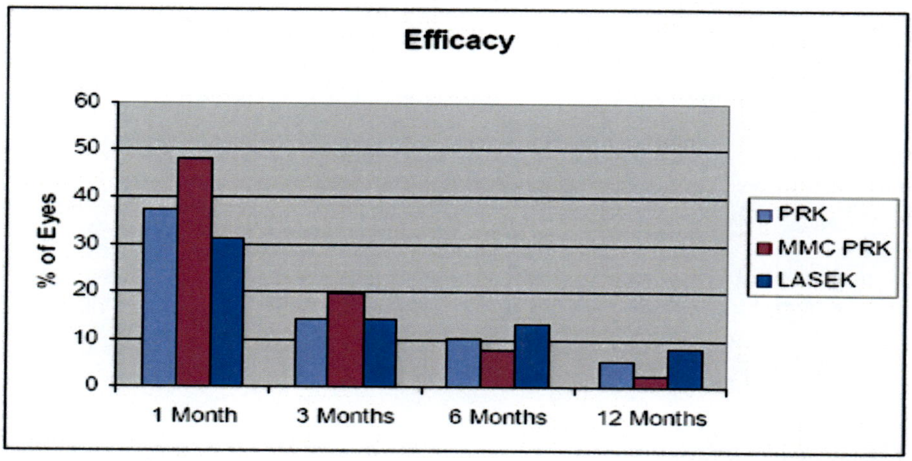


Figure 2. PreBSCVA vs PostUCVA eye with 2 or greater line loss.

# Predictability

Predictability was at 1, 3, 6 and 12 months. While there was a trend towards better predictability of MMC PRK compared to either PRK or LASEK at one and 6 months postoperatively, there was no difference between the groups at the 12 month postoperative visit (Table 1).

**Table 1. Predictability. Goal to emmetropia, percentage of eyes**

| | PRK | | MMC PRK | | LASEK | |
|---|---|---|---|---|---|---|
| | ±0.5D | ±1.0D | ±0.5D | ±1.0D | ±0.5D | ±1.0D |
| 1 Month | 44.8 | 73.3 | 56.6 | 84.3 | 46.3 | 76.8 |
| 3 Months | 57.3 | 80.0 | 58.3 | 86.1 | 58.4 | 79.2 |
| 6 Months | 64.9 | 85.5 | 82.5 | 92.1 | 69.1 | 82.4 |
| 12 Months | 81.5 | 96.7 | 86.4 | 95.5 | 81.6 | 91.7 |

**Table 2. Percentage of eyes with haze. No eye developed grade 3 or 4 haze. Grade 2 haze was only found in one LASEK eye at 1 month and 1 PRK eye at 6 and 12 months. All other haze was grade 1**

| | 1 Month | 3 Months | 6 Months | 12 Months |
|---|---|---|---|---|
| PRK | 13.3 | 10.7 | 7.7 | 5.4 |
| MMC PRK | 8.4 | 4.1 | 1.6 | 2.3 |
| LASEK | 25.6 | 19.3 | 7.4 | 4.2 |

# Quality of Vision

There were no statistically different changes between the three groups when measuring postoperative 5% LCVA and 25% LCVA. There was a trend towards improved 5% contrast in LASEK compared to PRK ($p = 0.096$) and MMC PRK ($p = 0.075$) at 3 months.

# Corneal Haze

At the one month preoperative visit, more haze was present in LASEK eyes compared to both PRK ($p = 0.021$) and MMC PRK ($p = 0.004$). The only eye that had haze of grade 2 was in the LASEK group. No eye in any group was grades 3 or 4. All other eyes were grade 1. LASEK continued to have a statistically significant increase in haze at 3 months compared to MMC PRK ($p = 0.005$), though no eyes at 3 months were grade 2 or higher. There was no statistical significance between groups at 6 or 12 months. One PRK eye at both 6 and 12 months had haze of grade 2, all other eyes in all groups with haze were grade 1. Total percentages of eyes with haze, both grades 1 and 2, can be seen in Table 2.

## Endothelial Cell Counts

Endothelial cell counts were done preoperatively and at 6 months and 12 months as a determinant of corneal health following refractive surgery. For the PRK group there was found to be a median loss of 37 cells/mm2 (range -1092 to 633) at 6 months postoperatively and 94 cells/mm2 (range -682 to 890) at 12 months. This change was statistically significant at 12 months (p – 0.001). For the MMC PRK group there was a median loss of 55 cells/mm2 (range -574 to 672) at 6 months and 35 cells/mm2 (-605 to 882) at 12 months, neither of which was statistically significant (p = -0.344 and 0.429 respectively). Additionally, there was no significant change for the LASEK group with a median loss of 17 cells/mm2 (range -936 to 546) at 6 months and a median gain of 37 cells/mm2 (range -789 to 791) at 12 months (p = 0.911 and 0.259 respectively). There was a significant difference between the 3 groups at 12 months (p = 0.021). This difference was found to be primarily between the PRK and LASEK groups (p = 0.004).

## EPI-LASIK Results at Walter Reed Army Medical Center

Another novel surface ablation technique, Epi-LASIK, was developed in an attempt to improve upon the advantages of LASEK. By using mechanical separation of the epithelium from the underlying corneal stroma, it is anticipated that the resulting cell morphology and physiology will be more normal when compared to the chemical separation method used in LASEK. Several preliminary studies have shown it to be a safe and efficient treatment. An ongoing study at Walter Reed Center for Refractive Surgery is in progress to determine the short and long term affects of this new procedure.

## Patients and Methods

A total of 290 eyes of 145 active duty US Army soldiers, age 21 or over, received bilateral Epi-LASIK using the Amadeus™ II epikeratome and LADARVision™ 6000 excimer laser system. Patients were treated for myopia or myopic astigmatism with a manifest refractive spherical equivalent between -0.5 to -6.25 diopters.

The epikeratome parameters were set per the manufacturer's recommendation. Once the flap was created, it was moved superiorly with use of a microspatula, and photoablation was done on the underlying stroma. If there was a complication in the first eye (right eye) a new epithelial separator was used for the second eye. The epithelial flap was retained after laser ablation whenever possible. After laser ablation the epithelial flap was replaced and a bandage contact lens was applied.

Preoperative data included age, gender MSE, refractive cylinder (CYL), keratometry (K) and central corneal thickness (CCT). Pain, corneal epithelium, UCVA and complications such as corneal infiltrates were assessed at 1 day, 4 days and 1 week postoperatively. UCVA,

BSCVA, MSE and 5% and 25% LCVA were assessed at 1, 3 and 6 month follow ups. The Epi-LASIK data were compared to an existing PRK data set that was collected under identical conditions.

Statistical analysis was performed using SPSS for Windows version 15.0. A Mann-Whitney test was used to compare UCVA and pain between Epi-LASIK and PRK. The Fisher's exact test was performed to assess the difference between the two groups when examining re-epithelialization and the presence of corneal infiltrates. A p-value of <0.05 was considered statistically significant. Odds ratios (OR) were used to determine likelihood of flap complications.

## Results

The mean age was 34 years old with 62.8% of patients male. The mean preoperative MSE was -2.93 +/- 1.19 D (range -1.00 to -6.25), mean cylinder was -0.56 +/- 0.51 D, K steep was 44.36 +/- 1.46 D, K flat was 43.55 +/- 1.44 D, and mean CCT was 540 +/- 34 µm.

## Intraoperative Complications

An overview of the intraopertative complications can be seen in **Table 3**. Overall, there was a 35% chance of a flap complication, with a 23% chance of losing the flap. There was a relative increase in rate of complications for age ≤40 (OR = 1.33, P = 0.022), CCT < 500 µm (OR = 1.227, P = 0.590), right eye (OR = 1.53, P = -.085), K cylinder >1.0D (OR = 1.33, P = 0.288), and K flat <42.0D (OR = 1.21, P = 0.568). There was a decreased odds ratio for K steep >46.0D (OR = 0.568, P = 0.160).

**Table 3. Epi-LASIK intraoperative flap complications, number of eyes and percentage**

| Complication | Number | Percent |
|---|---|---|
| No complication | 188 | 64.8 |
| Automatic flap amputation | 43 | 14.8 |
| Buttonhole flap | 17 | 5.9 |
| Hinge tear | 14 | 4.8 |
| Surgeon amputation (hinge in treatment zone) | 14 | 4.8 |
| Incomplete flap/ superficial resection | 8 | 2.8 |
| Stromal incursion | 6 | 2.1 |
| Total | 290 | 100.0 |

## Early Healing Results

There was no statistical difference in pain scores between Epi-LASIK and PRK at any visit in the first week postoperatively. Re-epithelialization was significantly faster in PRK eyes, with 92% of PRK eyes compared to only 55.4% of Epi-LASIK eye fully healed by postoperative day 4 ($p = 0.000$), and 99% of PRK eyes compared to 88.5% of Epi-LASIK eyes fully healed by postoperative day 7 ($p = 0.000$). A total of 50 Epi-LASIK eyes and no PRK eyes required an additional visit at postoperative day 10 to assess completion of re-epithelialization.

## Long Term Healing Results

Epi-LASIK was associated with significantly worse UCVA at postoperative day 1 ($p = 0.002$) when compared to PRK. Otherwise, there was no other significant difference in UCVA, BSCVA or MSE up to 6 months postoperatively over time between groups. Efficacy was evaluated by comparing preoperative BSCVA to postoperative UCVA. Up to 3 months there was no statistical significance between the two groups. At 6 months efficacy in epi-LASIK patients was significantly better than in PRK patients, with 83.9% of epi-LASIK patients attaining a postoperative UCVA the same or better than preoperative BSCVA compared to 71.7% of PRK patients. There was no statistical difference in haze formation at 1, 3 and 6 months. No eye developed grade 3 or 4 haze and only 2 Epi-LASIK eyes developed grade 2 haze at 1 month. All other haze at 1, 3 and 6 months was grade 1 haze.

## Discussion

Though LASIK has only shown an advantage over surface ablation techniques during the first few weeks postoperatively[77,78], those early healing benefits have caused LASIK to flourish. LASEK and Epi-LASIK were developed to incorporate those advantages to the safety profile seen in PRK.

As the primary purpose of refractive surgery is to obtain the best visual acuity possible without the use of spectacles, assessing the visual outcomes is a determining factor in the success of a technique. Comparing preoperative BSCVA with postoperative UCVA is likely the main factor that a patient uses to determine the success of refractive surgery. In our study, at one month eyes receiving LASEK had a significantly better outcome than eyes receiving MMC PRK, with a trend towards improvement compared to PRK. Visual acuity after 1 month was equivalent between all three groups. This is in contrast to the study done by Ghadfan et al.[79], which showed a slightly better outcome with the PRK techniques compared to LASEK. MMC PRK, however, showed better predictability compared to both PRK and LASEK at one month.

There has been concern for acoustic or ultraviolet radiation damage on corneal endothelial cell density, as well as cytotoxic effects of mitomycin-C. Previous studies have shown no adverse effect on the clinical endothelium, both without[80] and in the presence of mitomycin-C[81]. Our results showed only a significant decrease in eyes receiving PRK at 12 months. There was no difference in endothelial cell density in eyes receiving MMC PRK or LASEK.

Our Epi-LASIK results are as yet incomplete to determine long-term visual outcomes. Up to three months there appeared to be no difference compared to PRK though at 6 months Epi-LASIK showed better efficacy than PRK. However, there has been concern for intraoperative complications of the Epi-LASIK flap. Over one-third of all patients had a flap complication, with 23% of all patients loosing the flap. In addition, PRK eyes resulted in better postoperative healing, with faster re-epithelialization compared to Epi-LASIK eyes. Many patients that received Epi-LASIK also required an addition postoperative visit to assess healing and evaluate complications.

Haze has always been a concern in surface ablation procedures due to the loss of Bowman's layer and healing response. Previous studies have shown a decrease in haze in LASEK[82] and Epi-LASIK compared to PRK, our studies showed worsening haze with LASEK. Haze rate was comparable among Epi-LASIK eyes and PRK eyes, providing support that the increased haze in LASEK eyes may have been related to the ethanol rather than the presence of a flap. This haze, however, was clinically insignificant, with clinically significant haze equivalent in both PRK and LASEK eyes.

## Conclusion

Though the advent of LASIK surgery was thought to be the death knoll for PRK, new surface ablations techniques such as LASEK and Epi-LASIK, advanced laser systems and an effort to avoid lamellar flap complications have given new breath to this venerable procedure. Until such time that outcomes of one technique proves superior to the others, no one technique will replace the others. In the U.S. military, surface ablation procedures are the principle refractive technique as the complications involved with a lamellar flap are greater in this active population. Continued research into new methods of reducing haze formation, decreasing postoperative pain, and improving on the safety, efficacy and predictability of surface ablations techniques will produce superior visual outcomes.

## References

[1] Leo D. Bores, Refractive Eye Surgery, 2nd Ed. 2001 Blackwell Science, Inc. Malden Massachusetts. P. 6

[2] Donders FC. On the Anomalies of Accommodation and Refraction of the Eye [translated by William D. Moore, M.D.]. London: New Sydenham Society, 1864.

[3] Podolsky, M. Lawrence (1998) Cures Out of Chaos: How Unexpected Discoveries Led to Breakthroughs in Medicine and Health, Harwood Academic Publishers.

[4] AP Ferry, "Professor" Charles Tyrrell and his ideal sight restorer. *Ophthalmol.* 1986; 93:1246-57.

[5] Thornton SP. Background of incisional refractive surgery In: Wu HK, Thompson VM, et al, editors. Refractive Surgery New York: Thieme Medical Publishers, 1999:127–134.

[6] Lans LJ. Experimentelle Untersuchungen uber Entstehung von Astigmatismus durch night perforirende Corneawunden. *Arch. ophthalmol.* 1898; 45:117-152.

[7] Sato T. Treatment of conical cornea (incision of Descemet's membrane). *Acta Soc. Ophthalmol. Jpn* 1939; 43:544-555.

[8] Sato T, Akiyama K, Shibata H. A new surgical approach to myopia. *Am. J. Ophthalmol.* 1953; 36:823–829.

[9] Dawano H, Uesugi Y, Nakayasu K et al. Long-term follow up for bullous keratopathy after sato-type anterior-posterior corneal refractive surgery. *Am. J. Ophthalmol.* 2003; 136:1154-1155.

[10] Fyodorov SN, Durnev VV, Ivashina AI, Gudechkiv VB. Calculation method of effectiveness of anterior keratotomy in surgical correction of myopia. In Fyodorov SN (ed): Surgery for Anomalies in ocular Refraction. Moscow: The Moscow research institute for ocular Microsurgery. 1981, pp. 114-121.

[11] Krauss JM, Pauliafito CA steinert RF. Laser interactions with the cornea. *Surv. Ophthalmol.* 1986; 31:37-53.

[12] Seiler T. McDonnel PJ. Excimer laser photorefractive keratectomy. *Surv. Ophthalmol.* 1995; 40:89-118.

[13] Taboada J, Mikesell GW, Reed RD. Response of the corneal epithelium to KrF excimer laser pulses. Healthe phys 1981; 40:677-683.

[14] Trokel SL, Srinivasan R, Braren B. Excimer laser surgery of the cornea. *Am. J. Ophthalmol.* 1983; 96:710-715.

[15] Krueger RR, Trokel SL, Schubert HD. Interaction of ultraviolet laser light with the cornea. *Invest .Ophthalmol. Vis. Sci.* 1985; 26:1455-1464.

[16] Krueger RR, Trokel SL. Quantitation of corneal ablation by ultraviolet laser light. *Arch. ophthalmol.* 1985; 103:1741-1742.

[17] Keyes T, Clarke RH, Isner JM. Theory of photoablation and its implications for laser phototherapy. *J. Phys. Chem.* 1985; 89:4194-4196.

[18] Srinivasan R. Kinetics of ablative photodecompensation of organic polymers in the far-ultraviolet (193 nm). *J. Vac. Sci. Tech. B.* 1983; 1:923-926.

[19] Puliafito CA, Stern D, Drueger RR, et al. High-speed photography of excimer laser ablation of the cornea. *Arch. Ophthalmol.* 1987; 105:1255-1259

[20] Puliafito CA, Wong K, Steinert RF. Quantitative and ultrastructural studies of excimer laser ablation of the cornea at 193 and 248 nanometers. *Lasers Surg. Med.* 1987; 7:155-159.

[21] Barnes S, Azar DT. Excimer laser surface ablation: Photorefractive keratectomy (PRK) and laser subepithelial keratomileusis (LASEK). In: Smolin G, Foster CF, Azar DT, et al, eds. Smolin and Thoft's The Cornea: Scientific Foundations and Clinical Practice, 4th Ed. Philadelphia: Lippincott Williams and Wilkins 2005;1182-1199.

[22] Campos M, Trokel SL, McDonnell PJ. Surface morphology following photorefractive keratectomy. *Ophthalmic. Surg* .1993; 24:822-825.

[23] Unkroth A, Kleinschmidt J, Ziegler W, et al. Ablation of the cornea by using a low-energy excimer laser. *Graefes Arch Clin. Exp. Ophthalmol.* 1993; 231:303-307.

[24] Dougherty PJ, Wellish KL, Malony RK. Excimer laser ablation rate and corneal hydration. *Am. J. Ophthalmol.* 1994; 118:169-176.

[25] Seiler T, Wollensak J. In vivo experiments with the excimer laser – technical parameters and healing processes. Ophthalomologica 1986; 192:65-70.

[26] SeilerT, Wollensak J. Myopic photorefractive keratectomy with the excimer laser. One-year follow-up. *Ophthalmology* 1991; 98:1156-1163.

[27] L'Esperance FA, Taylor DM, Warner JW. Human excimer laser keratectomy: short-term histopathology. *Refract. Corneal Surg.* 1988; 96:654-664.

[28] O'Bart DPS, Corbett MC, Verma S, et al. Effects of ablation diameter, depth, and edge contour on the outcome of photorefractive keratectomy. *J. Refract. Surg.* 1996; 12:50-60.

[29] Kim J,Woo S, Park C, Hahn T, Kim M. Myopic regression after photorefractive keratectomy. *Ophthalmic. Surg .Lasers* 1996; 27:S435-439.

[30] Carson CA, Taylor HR. Excimer laser treatment for high and extreme myopia. *Arch. Ophthalmol.* 1995; 113:431–436.

[31] Braunstein RE, Jain S, McCally RI, et al. Objective measurement of corneal light scattering after excimer laser keratectomy. *Ophthalmol.* 1996; 103:439-443.

[32] Lin RT, Maloney RK. Flap complications associated with lamellar refractive surgery. *Am. J. Ophthalmol.* 1999; 127:129-136.

[33] Stulting DR, Carr JD, Thompson KP, et al. Complications of laser in situ keratomileusis for the correction of myopia. *Ophthalmol.* 1999; 106:13-20

[34] Al-Reefy M. Bacterial keratitis following laser in situ keratomileusis for hyperopia. *J. Refract. Surg*. 1999; 15:216-217.

[35] Wright JD Jr, Neubaur CC, Stevens G Jr. Epithelial ingrowth in a corneal graft treated by laser in situ keratuomileusis: light and electron microscopy. *J. Cataract Refract. Surg*. 2000; 26:49-55.

[36] Castillo A, Diaz-Valle D, Gutierrez AR, et. al. Peripheral melt of flap after laser in situ keratomileusis. *J. Refract. Surg.* 1998; 14:61-63.

[37] Lombardo AJ, Katz HR. Late partial dislocation of a laser in situ keratomileusis flap. *J. Cataract Refract. Surg* .2001; 27:1108-1110.

[38] Leung AT, Rao SK, Lam DS. Traumatic partial unfolding of laser in situ keratomileusis flap with severe epithelial ingrowth. *J. Cataract. Refract. Surg.* 2000; 26:135-139.

[39] Melki SA, Talamo JH, Demetriades Am, et al. Late traumatic dislocation of laser in situ keratomileusis corneal flap. *Ophthalmol* 2000; 107:2136-2139.

[40] Schwartz GS, Park DH, Schloff S, et al. Traumatic flap displacement and subsequent diffuse lamellar keratitis after laser in situ keratomileusis. *J. Cataract. Refract. Surg.* 2001; 27:781-783.

[41] Pallikaris IG, Kymionis GD, Astyrakakis NI. Corneal ectasia induced by laser in situ keratomileusis. *J. Cataract..Refract. Surg.* 2001; 27:1796-1802.

[42] Claringbold TV. Laser-assisted subepithelial keratectomy for the correction of myopia. J *Cataract. Refract. Surg*. 2002; 28:18-22.

[43] LeeJB, Ryu CH, Kim J, et al. Comparison of tear secretion and tear film instability after photorefractive keratectomy and laser in situ keratomileusis. *J. Cataract. Refract. Surg.* 2000 26:1326-1331.

[44] Kohnen T. Retreating residual refractive errors after excimer surgery of the cornea: PRK versus LASIK. *J. Cataract. Refract. Surg.* 2000;25:625-626.

[45] Sun R, Gimbel HV, Kaye GB. Photorefractive keratectomy in keratoconus suspects. J Cataract Refract Surg 1999; 25:1461-1466.

[46] Yo C, Vroman D, Ma S, et al. Surgical outcomes of photorefractive keratectomy and laser in situ keratomileusis by inexperienced surgeons. *J. Cataract. Refract. Surg.* 2000 ;26:510-515.

[47] Burka JM, Bower KS, VanRoekel RC, et al. The effect of moxifloxacin and gatifloxacin on long-term visual outcomes following photorefractive keratectomy. *J. Refract. Surg.* 2007; 23:414-417.

[48] Baldwin HC, Marshall J. Growth factors in corneal wound healing following refractive surgery: a review. *Acta Ophthalmol. Scand* 2002; 80:238-247.

[49] Li DG, Tseng SC. Three patterns of cytokine expression potentially involved in epithelial-fibroblast interactions of human ocular surface. *J. Cell Physiol.* 2000; 27:565-570.

[50] Moller-Peterson T. Keratocyte reflectivity and corneal haze. *Exp. Eye Res.* 2004; 78:553-560.

[51] Jester JV, Petroll WM, Cavanagh HD. Corneal stromal wound healing in refractive surgery: the role of myofibroblasts. *Prog. Retin Eye Res.* 1999; 18:311-356.

[52] Kaji Y, Obata H, usui T, et al. Three-dimensional organization of collagen fibrils during corneal stromal wound healing after excimer laser keratectomy. *J. Cataract Refract Surg.* 1998; 24:1441-1446.

[53] Jester JV, Moller-Pederson T, Huang J, et al. The cellular basis of corneal transparency: evidence for corneal crystallins. *J. Cell Sci.* 1999; 112:613-622.

[54] Mohan rr, Hutcheon AEK, Choi R, et al. Apoptosis, necrosis, proliferation, and myofibroblast generation in the stroma following LASIK and PRK. *Exp. Eye Res.* 2003; 76:71-87.

[55] Ambrosio R Jr, Wilson S. LASIK vs LASEK vs PRK: advantages and indications. Semin Ophthalmol 2003; 18:2-30.

[56] Gauthier CA, Holden BA, Epstein D, et al. Role of epithelial hyperplasia in regression following photorefractive keratectomy. *Br. J. Ophthalmol.* 1996; 80:545-548.

[57] Lohmann CP, Guell JL. Regression after LASIK for the treatment of myopia: the role of the epithelium. *Semin. Ophthalmol.* 1998; 13:79-82.

[58] Wilson SE, He Y-G, Weng J, et al. Effect of epidermal growth factor, hepatocyte grwoth factor, and keratinocyte frowth factor on proliferation, motility and differentiation of human corneal epithelial cells. *Exp. Eye. Res.* 1994; 59:665-78.

[59] Choi SY, Kim HY, Kim JY, et al. Two-year follow-up of eyes without topical corticosteroid treatment after photorefractive keratectomy (PRK). *Korean J. Ophthalmol.* 1998; 12:25-29.

[60] Corbett MC, O'Bart DP, Marshall J. Do topical corticosteroids have a role following excimer laser photorefractive keratectomy? *J. Refract. Surg.* 1995; 11:380-387.

[61] Gartry DS, Kerr Muir M, Marshall J. The effect of topical corticosteroids on refraction and corneal haze following excimer laser treatment of myopia: an update. A prospective, randomized, double-masked study. *Eye* 1993; 7:584-590.

[62] Vigo L, Scandola E, Carones F. Scraping and mitomycin C to treat haze and regression after photorefractive keratectomy for myopia. *J. Refract. Surg.* 2003; 19:449-454.

[63] Raviv T, Majmudar PA, Dennis RF, et al. Mitomycin-C for post-PRK corneal haze. *J. Cataract. Refract .Surg.* 2000; 26:1105-1106.

[64] Carones F, Vigo L, Scandola E, et al. Evaluation of the prophylatice use of mitomycin-C to inhibit haze formation after photorefractive keratectomy. *J. Cataract. Refract. Surg.* 2002; 28:2088-2095.

[65] Kasetsuwan N, Wu FM, Hsieh F, et al. Effect of topical ascorbic acid on free radical tissue damage and inflammatory cell influx in the corneal after excimer laser corneal surgery. *Arch. Ophthalmol.* 1999; 117:649-652.

[66] Stojanovic A, Ringvold A, Nitter T. Ascorbate prophylaxis for corneal haze after photorefractive keratectomy. *J. Refract Surg.* 2003; 19:338-343.

[67] Anderson Penno E, Braun DA, Kamal A, et al. Topical thiotepa treatment for recurrent corneal haze after photorefractive keratectomy. *J. Cataract. Refract. Surg.* 2003; 29:1537-1542.

[68] Camellin M, Cimberle M. LASEK technique promising after 1 year of experience. Ocul Surg News 2000; 18:14-17.

[69] Lee JB, Seong GJ, Lee JH et al. Comparison of laser epithelial keratomileusis and photorefractive keratectomy for low to moderate myopia. *J. Cataract. Refract. Surg.* 2001; 27:565-570.

[70] Azar CT, Ang RT. Laser subepithelial keratomileusis: evolution of alcohol assisted flap surface ablation. *Int. Ophthalmol. Clin.* 2002; 42:89-97.

[71] Vinciguerra P, Camesasca FL. Butterfly laser epithelial keratomileusis for myopia. *J. Refract. Surg.* 2002; 18(3 Suppl):S371-S373.

[72] Samalonies LB. Gel-assisted LASEK. Eyeworld. February 2002. Available at: http://www.eyeworld.org/article.php?sid=2201. Accessed Feb 8, 2008.

[73] Chen CC, Change JH, Lee JB et al. Human corneal epithelial cell viability and morphology after dilute alcohol exposure. *Invest. Oophthalmol. Vis. Sci.* 2002; 43:2593-602.

[74] Pallikaris IG, Katsanevaki VJ, Kalyvianaki MI, et al. Advances in subepithelial excimer refractive surgery techniques: Epi-LASIK. Curr. *Opin. Ophthalmol.* 2003; 14:207-212.

[75] Pallikaris IG, Katsanevaki VJ, Kalyvianaki MI, et al. Epi-LASIK: comparative histological evaluation of mechanical and alcohol-assisted epithelial separation. *J. Cataract. Refract. Surg.* 2003; 29;1496-1501.

[76] Hammond MD, Madigan WP, Bower KS. Refractive Surgery in the US Army: 2000 – 2003. *Ophthalmology* 2005 Feb;112:184-190.)

[77] Pop M, Payette Y. Photorefractive keratectomy versus laser in situ keratomileusis. *Ophthalmol.* 2000; 107:251-257.

[78] El Danasoury MC, Maghraby AE, Elyce SD et al. Comparison of photorefractive keratectomy with excimer laser in situ keratomileusis in correcting low myopia (from -2.00 to -5.50 diopters). A randomized study. *Ophthalmol* 1999; 106:411-421.

[79] Ghadfan F, Al;Rajhi A, Wagoner MD. Laser in situ keratomileusis versus surface ablation: Visual outcomes and complications. *J. Cataract. refract.* Surg 2007; 33:2041-2048.

[80] Jabbur NS. Endothelial cell studies in patients after photorefractive keratectomy for hyperopia. *J. Refract. Surg.* 2003; 19:142-148.

[81] Diakonis VF, Pallikaris A, Kymionis GD, et al. Alterations in endothelial cell density after photorefractive keratectomy with adjuvant mitomycin. *Am. J. Ophthalmol.* 2007; 144:99-103.

[82] Shah S, Sebai Sarhan AR, Doyle SJ, et al. The epithelial flap for photorefractive keratectomy. *Br. J. Ophthalmol.* 2001; 85:393-396.

In: Laser Keratectomy: Approaches, Complications...
Author: Luis W. Schröder and Felix J. Walter
ISBN 978-1-60456-863-9


*Chapter II*

# Corneal Refractive Surgery with Laser: Safety and Effectiveness

***Raúl Martín Herranz****
IOBA Eye Institute, Avda. del Cementerio s/n (Campus Miguel Delibes).
47011 Valladolid, Spain

## Abstract

Different corneal refractive procedures are used to correct ametropias. In the 1950's, Barraquer described the first corneal procedures with corneal keratomileusis to correct low, moderate and high myopia and hyperopia. In the 1970's, Fyodorov and Durnev described radial keratectomy to correct myopia. In the 1980's, Trokel described the use of the excimer laser in refractive corneal surgery with Photorefractive Keratectomy (PRK), and at the end of the decade McDonald and Pallikaris described Laser-Assisted in Situ Keratomileusis (LASIK). Today, laser procedures are the most frequent corneal refractive surgeries, with techniques such as Photorefractive Keratectomy (PRK), Laser-Assisted in-situ Keratomileusis (LASIK) and Wavefront-guided LASIK, and Conductive keratoplasty (CK).

Photorefractive Keratectomy (PRK) applies excimer laser ablation directly to the Bowman membrane after corneal des-epithelisation. This technique is safe and effective for correcting low ametropias (lower than 6.00 D).

Laser-Assisted in-situ Keratomileusis (LASIK) applies excimer laser ablation to the stroma after making a corneal flap. It is safe and effective for correcting low and moderate myopia and low hyperopia with or without moderate astigmatism. Different software makes it possible to correct optical aberrations of the eye, such as coma, spherical aberration and others, with wave-front guided LASIK.

More recently, Conductive Keratoplasty (CK) using a holmium laser has been approved by the FDA to correct low hyperopia and presbyopia. This procedure applies a holmium laser to the corneal periphery to steepen the corneal curvature.

* Tel: +34 983 423559, +34 983 423260, FAX: 983 423723, Email: raul@ioba.med.uva.es.

In last two decades, some research has been carried out to verify the safety and efficacy of these different surgical techniques, and to determine the patients' degree of satisfaction.

The purpose of this chapter is to describe the main characteristics, surgical procedures, indications, effectiveness, efficacy, predictability, complications, secondary effects and long-term effects of these corneal laser keratectomy procedures.

## Introduction

Refractive Surgery (RS) is defined[1] as "modifying the refraction of the eye through surgery", and may be carried out at corneal level – *known as corneal refractive surgery* – and at *intraocular* level, implanting intraocular lenses (IOL) with or without extraction of the clear lens[2].

Corneal refractive surgery techniques are possible due to the cornea being a flexible, elastic medium, capable of changing shape, and with the highest refractive power of the eyeball (40-45 dioptres). It is also a type of tissue with a "memory", meaning it tends to return to its original shape after a trauma or surgery. This quality defines the unpredictable nature of the results of refractive surgery in a particular patient[3].

## Indications for Performing Refractive Surgery

Refractive surgery may be indicated for persons who have an intolerance to conventional methods for correcting ametropias, whether glasses or contact lenses, as well as for those who need to improve their VA without glasses or contact lenses, reducing their dependency on a compensation system or using slimmer and more aesthetic lenses, for example, for reasons connected with their type of work[1-3].

Persons at ages close to presbyopia are not ideal candidates for refractive surgery, as the techniques used to correct it do not offer the same results as those used for correcting myopia; however, the appearance of new designs of multifocal intraocular lenses is achieving highly promising results in correcting this type of refractive defect, as we will see later in this article.

## Outcomes in Refractive Surgery

In order to objectively evaluate the results of any refractive surgery procedure, it is important to know how its safety, efficacy, predictability and stability are defined [4-6].

*Safety* is defined in this case as the incidence and severity of the complications associated with a procedure. This index is established by calculating the loss of two or more lines of best-corrected visual acuity (BCVA) after surgery. It is calculated mathematically by defining the quotient between the uncorrected visual acuity (UCVA) and VA with previous correction. A loss of 2 or more lines of VA by 5% is considered unacceptable.

*Efficacy* is determined by the number of eyes that achieve UCVA after surgery equivalent to 20/40 or higher on the Snellen scale.

**Table 1. Indices used to evaluate the results of different refractive surgery techniques.**

| | |
|---|---|
| Safety | $\frac{Postoperative\ BCVC}{Preoperative\ BCVA}$ Percentage of the loss of 2 or more lines of VA |
| Efficacy | N° of eyes with UCVA ≥20/40 (Snellen scale) |
| Predictability | Percentage of eyes with ±1.00 D or ±0.50 D |
| Stability | Changes in postoperative refraction |

This is the minimum VA required to obtain a driving permit in many countries (such as Spain or the USA). The main goal of refractive surgery is to reduce or eliminate dependency on glasses or contact lenses, and does not have to imply achieving "perfect" vision after surgery.

*Predictability* is defined as the probability of the surgical procedure achieving the required correction, normally refractive emmetropia. It is determined by the percentage of eyes with a spherical equivalent refraction (SER) of between ±1.00 D and ±0.50 D after surgery.

Finally, *stability* refers to refractive changes within a given period of time after surgery

# Surgical Techniques

There are numerous surgical techniques for the treatment of refractive errors, described since the mid-twentieth century (with the first surgical techniques for myopia dating from the eighteenth century). However, only a few have achieved levels of efficacy and safety that may be considered acceptable in clinical terms. The most typical are Radial Keratotomy, Photorefractive Keratotomy (PRK) and Laser-assisted in-situ Keratomileusis (LASIK). Other increasingly popular methods are intraocular refractive surgery (mainly for cases outside of the range of LASIK), and conductive keratoplasty (CK) for hyperopia and presbyopia. Other techniques include intraocular lens (IOL) implants, with or without extraction of the clear lens, which are an alternative for important refractive errors, and to correct presbyopia[7].

## Radial Keratotomy (RK)

Dr. Sato developed the origins of this Technique in Japan between 1939 and 1953, making incisions in the frontal and posterior surface of the cornea. Dr. Yenaliev modified the procedure between 1969 and 1978, with incisions only in the frontal surface. In Russia in the 1970's, Doctors Fyodorov and Durnev described RK as it is known today, publishing their results in 1979. Dr. Bores introduced RK into the USA for the first time in 1978. Dr. Ruiz observed that by varying the pattern of the incisions, it was also possible to compensate astigmatism[8].

RK is based on relaxing the connective mesh of the corneal tissue, with the surgeon making very deep radial incisions with a scalpel to between 80-90% of the thickness of the cornea. These incisions leave a fine, whitish scar, and extend radially (Figure 1).

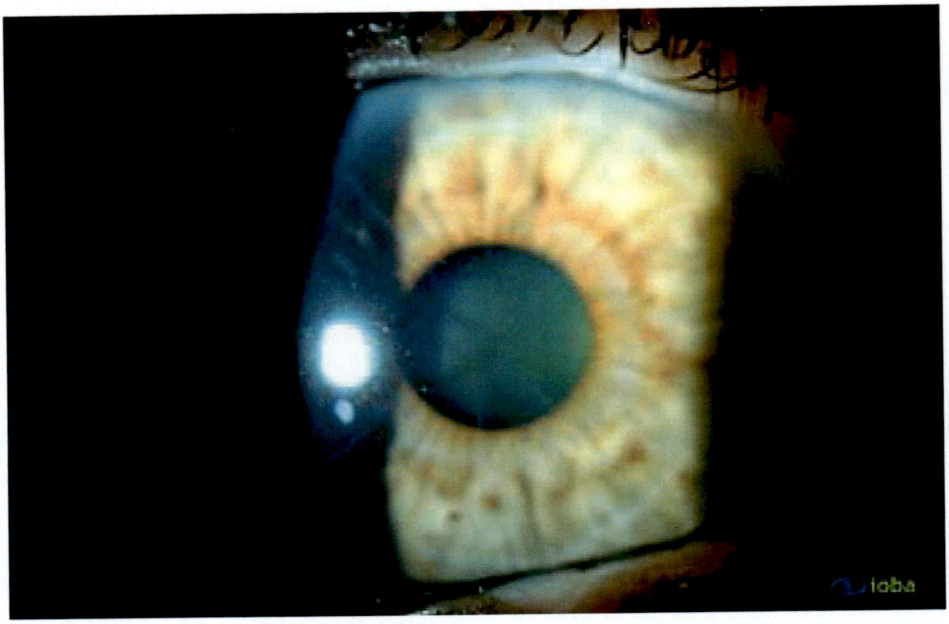


Figure 1. Detail of an eye operated on using radial keratotomy. The radial cuts (white lines) may be seen in the cornea, extending beyond the pupillary diameter.

This technique has been supplanted by laser surgery, mainly as a result of its complications (the risk of corneal perforation during surgery, the structural "weakening" of the eyeball and progressive hypermetropisation), as demonstrated in the Prospective Evaluation of Radial Keratotomy (PERK) study in 19949 after 10 years of follow. However, due to its low cost, it is one of the most frequently performed surgical techniques in the world. Other authors have proposed its use for treating serious astigmatism (full-arc incisions10) either as a stand-alone procedure or combined with other techniques such as LASIK[11].

## Photorefractive Keratectomy (PRK)

Excimer laser technology is based on combining two gases (one noble gas and a halogen). The wavelength obtained depends on the gases used: if argon and fluorine are combined, a wavelength of 193 nm is emitted, in the ultraviolet spectrum and highly effective for corneal surgery, as it produces a more precise, even cut, causing less thermal and acoustic damage to adjacent tissue.

The interaction of the photons from the laser beam with the tissues produces a breakdown in the molecular bonds and the resulting loss of tissue. This process is known as photoablation[1,2,12,13].

The excimer laser started to be used in the treatment of ametropias in the 1980's, with Dr. Trokel publishing the first articles on experiments using the technique[14]. The first applications for the laser were to make the cuts used in RK, avoiding the use of scalpels and the associated complications. In April 1996 the FDA[15] approved the use of 2 excimer lasers to carry out photorefractive and phototherapeutic keratotomies in the USA. Subsequently, the excimer laser would be applied intrastromally, leading to the LASIK technique.

This surgical technique may be appropriate for patients who meet the following requirements:

- Slight or moderate myopia, less than -6.00 D.
- Moderate hypermetropia, less than +4.00 D.
- Slight or moderate astigmatism, less than 4.50 D.
- Stable refraction.
- Intolerance to using contact lenses, and impossibility or unwillingness to use corrective glasses (for psychological or professional reasons).

This technique is performed by applying the laser directly to Bowman's membrane, after removing the corneal epithelium either mechanically or chemically. This causes discomfort in the postoperative period for the patient as it causes a large corneal ulcer (the size of the area treated with the laser), which may cause moderate to severe pain, requiring treatment with analgesics.

The most frequent complication involved in PRK is the appearance of an opaque corneal opacity scar or 'haze' (figure 2). This opacity is found in 92% of cases, although it is only significant (leading to a decrease in the VA or other symptoms) in 1%. A higher level of haze is associated with the higher the ametropias being treated, the deeper the ablation, the more heterogeneous the laser beam during surgery, and other intrapersonal motives, although there is no clearly accepted consensus.

Other complications of PRK surgery (which it shares with LASIK surgery, as both are refractive processes using excimer lasers, although with different rates of prevalence) include refractive regression (evolution of the refractive result that remains within the pre-surgical refraction range, estimated to be from 9% in myopias from -3 to -6 D to 20% in myopias from -6 to -9 D), decreased VA (from 1% in myopias of less than 6 D to 7% in higher myopias), decreased contrast sensitivity (from 5% to 20% in the early post-operative period), halos, dazzling and problems with night vision (5% to 50% of people who have been operated on refer to increased dazzling and problems with night vision), hyper- or hypocorrection, unstable refraction, induced astigmatism, decentring, central islands and other less frequent complications.

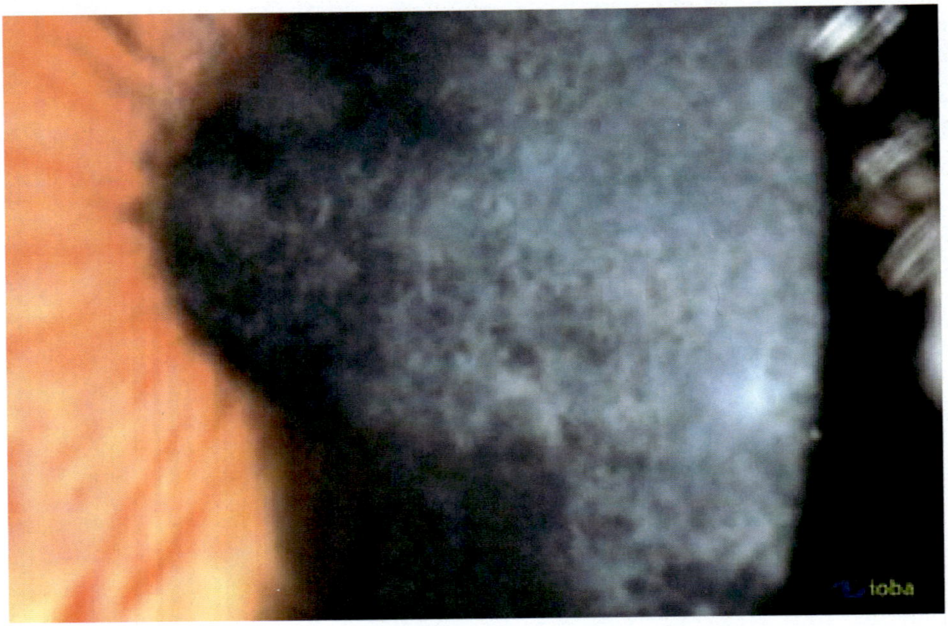


Figure 2. Corneal haze. The scar in the shape of a small square cloudy patch may be seen, with the typical greyish-white colour of post-PRK corneal haze. The maximum AV after surgery was 20/50 on the Snellen scale.

A variant of this technique involves removing the corneal epithelium, carrying out the laser ablation and replacing the epithelium in its original position. This technique is known as de laser-assisted subepithelial keratectomy (LASEK)[16,17]. It permits better results than the PRK technique18,19 in terms of postoperative pain and discomfort, with faster visual recovery and less corneal haze, leading to a less intense scarring process [20] with better refractive results, and less complications in the treatment of moderate myopia (between -1.50 and -7.50 D). Compared to the LASIK technique, LASEK avoids the complications caused by making a corneal flap[16,17], with similar visual and refractive results. However, the visual recovery process is slower[21] and has a higher tendency towards overcorrection[22] in the treatment of low and moderate myopia. The LASEK technique has also been proposed for the treatment of moderate hypermetropia (less than +5.00 D) with good refractive and visual results[23].

## Laser-Assisted in Situ Keratomileusis (LASIK)

LASIK is the acronym for Laser-Assisted in Situ Keratomileusis, which is possibly the most widely used surgical technique and the most in demand from wearers of glasses and/or contact lenses.

This technique was proposed by Dr. M. McDonald in 1987 [24,25] and Dr. Pallikaris[26-28], making use of the work of Dr. Barraquer, who developed the first microkeratome in the mid-1950's. The main advantage of the LASIK technique is that the epithelium and Bowman's membrane remain virtually intact[29]. This reduces the haze and myopic regression seen in patients who undergo PRK, achieving higher visual sharpness without correction more quickly, a more regular corneal topography, and reducing postoperative pain and discomfort[30].

The LASIK technique was approved by the FDA for treating ametropias in July 1999 (www.fda.gov ).[13]

**Table 2. Summary of the data for efficacy, stability and safety used by the FDA to approve the LASIK technique. *Types of Excimer laser**

| | Summit * | Visx * |
|---|---|---|
| Eyes | 1013 | 723 |
| Efficacy | | |
| UCVA ≥ 20/40 post LASIK | 92% | 95% |
| UCVA ≥ 20/20 | | |
| Pre-op myopia < 7.00 D | 51% | 63% |
| Pre-op myopia > 7.00 D | 29% | 39% |
| Manifest refraction | | |
| ≤ 0.50 D | 61% | 75% |
| ≤ 1.00 D | 84% | 91% |
| Stability | | |
| Change < 1.00 D at 3-6 months | 94% | 95% |
| Safety | | |
| Loss of 2 or more lines of VA | 1.9% | 0.6% |
| Induced astigmatism | 1% | 0% |
| Adverse effects | <1% | <1% |

The main indications for LASIK surgery are:

- Myopias from -1.00 D to -10.00 D (up to -5.00 D it offers refractive results similar to PRK). There is no widely accepted consensus on the upper limit of dioptres, mainly depending on the anatomical factors (corneal thickness) of the patient and the laser used during surgery.
- Astigmatisms up to 6.00 D.
- Hypermetropias up to +8.00 D.
- Stable refraction.

On the contrary, patients with the following indications are not good candidates:

- Slight or moderate ametropia.
- Ocular pathology, especially anterior pathologies.
- Chronic ophthalmic pathology (such as glaucoma).
- Corneas with reduced thickness, which do not permit a post-surgical corneal thickness of at least 400 micras.

- Systemic pathology: diabetes (a relative contraindication with good metabolic control[31]), autoimmune pathology (systemic lupus erythematosus, rheumatoid arthritis, etc.) and pregnancy.
- Psychological indications (non-realistic expectations of the surgery).

The surgical technique involves making a cut in a fine corneal layer that includes the epithelium, Bowman's membrane and several micras of the anterior stroma. This layer is referred to as the corneal flap. In order to cut the flap, an instrument known as a microkeratome is required. Laser systems are also available (femtosecond lasers) to avoid the complications derived from using the microkeratome[32-34].

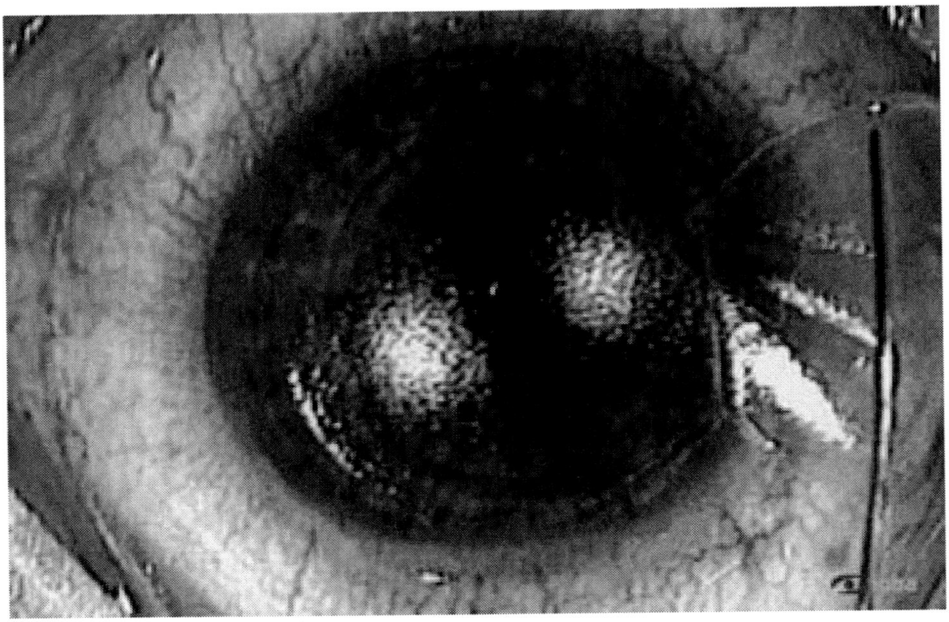

Figure 3. Detail of the surgical process during LASIK surgery. The corneal flap may be seen to the right, with the stromal stratum ready to apply laser ablation to the stromal surface.

During surgery, the intraocular pressure must be raised above 60 mmHg in order to cut the flap efficiently with the microkeratome. Once the cut has been made, the flap is lifted and the excimer laser is applied to the stromal surface (figure 3).

The results of the LASIK technique for correcting myopia make it possible to obtain a post operatory refraction of ±1.00 D in between 85% and 96% of patients, and ±0.50 D for between 75% and 90% in a safe, effective manner, without any loss of VA. These results are related to the previous ametropia of the patient[35].

The LASIK technique for treating moderate hypermetropia (less than +5.00 D) has a safety index of 0.90, with a loss of lines of vision of less than 2%. Between 80% and 90% of cases have an uncorrected VA of 20/40 or higher, and between 45% and 60% of 1.0 or higher. The refractive error after surgery is +1.00 D for between 80% and 90%, and ±0.50D for 60%[35-37]. Furthermore, in the case of hypermetropia surgery, there is a higher prevalence of regression than that found for myopia surgery[36,37] and a higher risk of losing visual sharpness in patients with post operatory hypermetropia higher than +5.00 D[38]. It has also been connected with a higher risk of having epithelial defects with age (patients over the age of 40) and in hypermetropic patients[39].

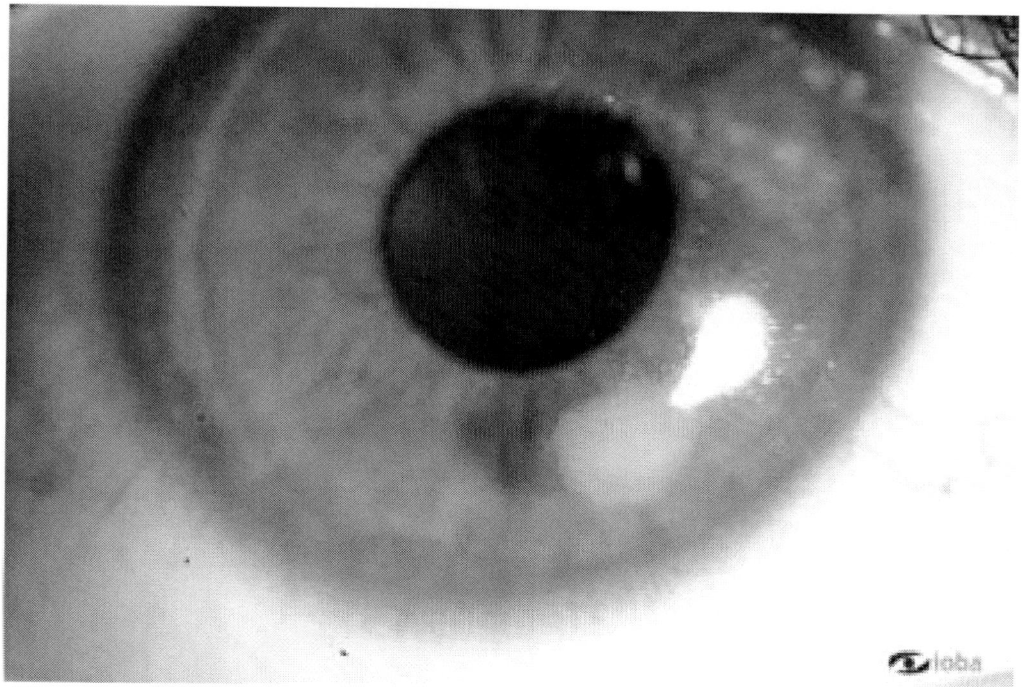

Figure 4. Growth of epithelial cells beneath the flap. These form an irregular, whitish grey deposit under the corneal flap.

**Table 2. Summary of the main complications of the LASIK technique [45-58]**

| | | |
|---|---|---|
| Intraoperative complications (1-2%) | Loss of suction | 0.30 % |
| | Incomplete Flaps | 0.30 % |
| | Buttonholes | 0.30 % |
| | Destructured Flap | 0.10 % |
| | Flap dislocation | 0.10 % |
| Early complications (within 48h) (<3.0 %) | Flap repositioning | 0.10 % |
| | Flap folds or stretching | 0.30 % |
| | Diffuse lamellar keratitis (DLK) | 2.30 % |
| | Infectious keratitis | 0.04 % |
| Later complications (after 48h) | Epithelial ingrowth | 10- 40 % |
| | Flap melting (> 0.5mm) | 0.36 % |
| | Decentring (>1mm) | 2.00 % |
| | Dry eye symptoms | 55.00 % |
| | Night vision problems | 5 to 50 % |

Unfortunately, like all surgical procedures, LASIK surgery suffers from a series of particular complications. Along with PRK surgery (as both processes require the use of an excimer laser), it shares the problems associated with the application of the laser, combined with those derived from the need to cut the flap (such as problems during suction, irregular or complete cuts, buttonholes, etc.), interstitial keratitis, corneal melting, epithelial ingrowth (figure 4), folds or striae in the flap (figure 5), etcetera, although these occur in a very low percentage (lower than 2-3%). Cases have also been described of the flap becoming dislocated several years after surgery as a result of mild traumas or injuries caused by airbags [40-43].

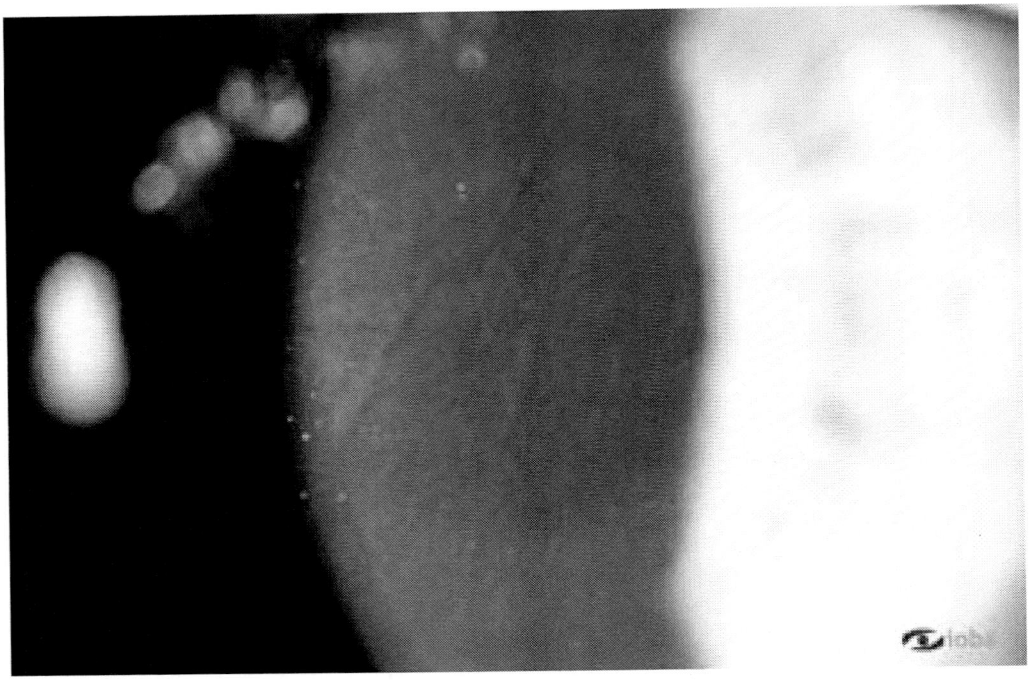

Figure 5. Detail of 'pleats' in the flap of a patient treated with LASIK. The pleats stand out as darker lines in the pupillary area.

Perhaps the most frequent complications are problems with night vision, which may affect between 5% and 50% of patients operated on using LASIK [44].

The complications involved may be classified chronologically, as intraoperative complications, early complications (within 48 hours), or later complications (after 48 hours) (see Table 2).

Finally, LASIK surgery presents two problems that are still unresolved; firstly, the corneal ablation (myopic or hypermetropic) induces high order optical aberrations, decreasing the quality of the eye as an optical instrument[59-62], degrading the retinal image; and secondly, there is no clear definition or consensus on the correct minimum corneal thickness following surgery to permit adequate biomechanical stability of the cornea, preventing the appearance of post-LASIK corneal ectasia[63-66].

In order to solve the first problem (inducing aberrations), different types of software have been developed for use with the laser, aimed at improving the ablated corneal surface, known as Custom Wavefront LASIK Eye Surgery[67]. The use of this software makes it possible to slightly improve the refractive result of conventional LASIK surgery[68-70]. A relation has also been found between the microkeratome used during surgery and the high level optical aberrations induced after surgery[71], although this relationship has not been clearly defined[72]. Some studies have also detected an increase in ocular aberrations even after carrying out custom wavefront LASIK eye surgery[73-76].

This loss of optical quality in the eye leads to the degradation of the retinal image, which together with the difference between the pupillary diameter and the diameter of the ablation, may justify the appearance of problems with vision, especially in conditions of scotopic vision, referred to by between 5% and 50% of patients who undergo LASIK surgery, indicating the presence of glare, dazzling and halos, which seriously impair night vision and activities such as driving.

The second unresolved problem, the appearance of corneal ectasia post-surgery which behaves in the same way as keratoconus (a corneal pathology characterised by the progressive thinning of the cornea, generally around the rim), has been identified thanks to the incorporation of high-tech methods applied to studying corneal topography (elevation topography making it possible to measure the curvature of the anterior and posterior corneal surfaces). The appearance of ectasia is related to the depth of the laser ablation (the quantity of dioptres operated on) and the diameter of the ablation. However, no techniques exist that make it possible to previously identify a patient who will develop a post-LASIK ectasia[77,78] suspecting the presence of factors, some of which are known (high myopia, keratoconus fustrum and low residual stromal bed thickness) and others that are unknown, which may affect the biomechanical stability of the cornea[79]. More extensive studies are required that define the incidence and prevalence of this complication, its detection prior to surgery, surgical criteria for safety, diagnostic criteria, etcetera, as there are numbers of patients with high myopias who have not developed posterior corneal ectasia after LASIK.

Myopic patients operated on using the LASIK have a very high level of satisfaction with the results of the surgery (with more than 90% declaring they are satisfied or very satisfied, and would undergo surgery again). However, 33% of these patients consider that their night vision is worse or much worse following surgery[44]. Furthermore, around 50% refer to suffering from more glare that reduces their vision after surgery, than previously with their glasses or contact lenses. With regard to driving, 60% of patients refer to the glare caused by vehicle headlights, and 40% refer to other problems when driving at night.

Some studies have not detected any relation between glare and night driving problems with the level of correction, the depth of the ablation or differences between the diameter of the pupil and the ablation. Other authors have suggested that these problems are related to the degradation of the retinal image (increased anomalies) presented by patients who have been operated on for myopia by LASIK.

## Conductive Keratoplasty (CK)

Conductive keratoplasty[80,81] uses a Holmium laser to reduce the corneal curvature, increasing its dioptric potential so that the hypermetropic refraction decreases. This is based on the retraction of collagen caused by the burn from the laser applied to the corneal periphery at approximately 6.0 and 7.0 mm (Figure 6).

This method is indicated [82,83] for the treatment of moderate hypermetropia and presbyopia in patients over the age of 40 with refractive errors of between +0.75 D and +3.25 D of hypermetropia, with less than -0.75 D of astigmatism (negative), and with a difference of more than 0.50 D between pre-surgical refraction with or without cyclopegic drugs.

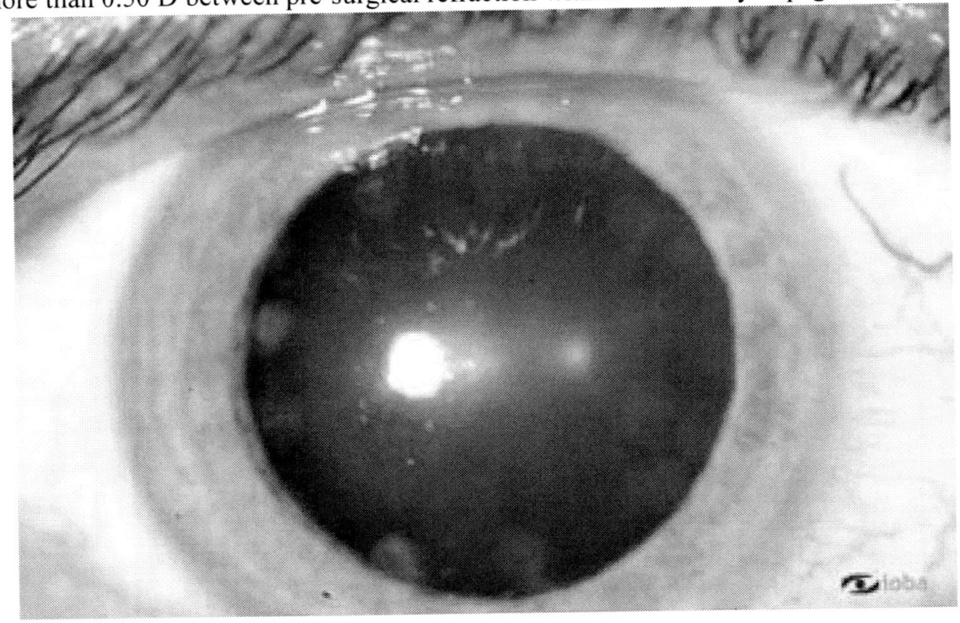

Figure 6. Conductive Keratoplasty for hypermetropia and presbyopia. The peripheral leukomas may be seen, which contract the collagen in order to increase the refractive capacity of the cornea.

It is contraindicated in patients with corneal pachymetry (at 6 mm peripherally) of less than 560 micras, previous surgery for strabismus, a history of herpetic keratitis, systemic illnesses (diabetes, autoimmune pathology, collagen pathology, atopic illnesses, immunosuppression, treatment with corticoids, or a history of keloid scarring), chronic dry eye syndrome or keratoconus.

The results presented by the FDA (www.fda.gov, 2002) conclude that it is a safe and effective technique for correcting hypermetropia, achieving an uncorrected VA of 20/20 for between 51% and 84% of patients one year after surgery, and higher than 20/40 for between 91% and 100%. Postoperative refraction is in the range of ±0.50 D for between 60% and 90% in ±1.00 D for between 91% and 100%. In terms of safety, less than 1% of patients lose 2 lines of VA, and an increase in the astigmatism (by more than 2.00 D) in less than 1% of cases.

Problems with night vision are classified as severe in 3% of cases, noticeable in 6% and moderate in 8% (representing a total of 17% with moderate to severe night vision problems). There is also a tendency towards regression 2 years after surgery[84].

## Intraocular Surgery

Intraocular surgery is classified in two categories, depending on whether the clear lens is removed, or if an intraocular lens (IOL) is fitted, maintaining the patient's clear lens and their accommodation capacity. In this second case, the IOL may be fitted in the anterior chamber (in front of the iris), or in the posterior chamber (between the iris and the clear lens)[85].

## Clear Lens Extraction (CLE)

This is the surgical alternative for correcting high ametropias[86]. Problems such as posterior capsular opacification, retinal detachment and macular edema are more prevalent in the case of high myopias or in young individuals, although the same complications may be expected as with cataract surgery. A higher rate of retinal detachment than would be expected has been referred to in the literature for patients with high myopias who have not undergone surgery[87], although other studies did not find any increase in this complication[88].

This technique has proved to be effective, with an acceptable predictability and few complications in patients with high myopia[89,90]. The choice to implant an interocular lens also makes it possible to correct presbyopia if a multifocal IOL is used[91].

## Anterior Chamber Intraocular Lenses

There are several types of interocular lenses used to correct high myopia, including the Baikoff or angular support lens, and the Worst-Fechner or iridian support lens, which are proposed as alternatives for correcting high myopia[92-94]. Although the optical results seem to be similar, both lenses induce a loss of endothelial cells, chronic inflammation and night halos, depending on the size of the patient's pupil; furthermore, iridian support lenses may also deform the pupil[95,96].

## Posterior Chamber Intraocular Lenses

In 1986, Fyodorov published the first description of this type of lens, using silicone IOL. Some authors consider this technique as being the main alternative to LASIK to maintain the accommodation capacity[97,98] proposing that it should also be used to correct astigmatism[99]. Its main complications include inducing cataracts as a result of the IOL rubbing against the clear lens, a loss of endothelial cells, chronic anterior uveitis[100] and acute closed angle glaucoma [101].

A combination of several techniques has been proposed for individuals with myopias and hypermetropias who are not candidates for LASIK surgery, such as implanting an IOL followed by LASIK to eliminate the residual refractive defect[102].

The use of multifocal IOLs offers a safe and effective alternative to the surgical correction of presbyopia, with good refractive results and for near- and far-sightedness comparable to those obtained in the treatment of myopia or hypermetropia[91,103,104], with multiple designs of IOLs (aspherical, diffractive, pseudo-accommodative, etc.) with different results[105,106]. These present a series of inconveniences, including the loss of visual sharpness in intermediate vision[107], decreased sensitivity to contrast[108,109], halos and nocturnal glare[110,111], dependency of the pupillary diameter (improved vision with pupils less than 3.0 mm in diameter)[112] and a possibly increased risk of opacification of the lens compared to patients with implants of monofocal IOLs[113].

## Conclusions

Different surgical techniques exist for the correction of ametropias (Table 3), which may act at corneal and/or intraocular level (LIO implant). The most popular and widespread technique for correcting myopia and hypermetropia with or without astigmatism is LASIK surgery, either on its own or combined with other techniques, such as incisive surgery when there is moderate astigmatism. Intraocular surgical techniques are indicated for the correction of strong ametropias, maintaining or removing the clear lens depending on the patient's age, ocular morphology and surgical technique to be used. In turn, conductive thermokeratoplasty is also proposed for correcting moderate hypermetropia and presbyopia (mainly with the monovision technique). Finally, promising results are being obtained for the correction of presbyopia with new designs of multifocal intraocular lenses.

**Table 3. Summary of the alternatives available for correcting ametropias. CL = Contact Lenses**

| Type of Ametropia | Strength (D) | Surgical Correction | Optical correction |
|---|---|---|---|
| Myopia | 0.00 to −1.00<br>−1.25 to −5.00<br>−5.25 to −12.00<br>> −12.25 | Not indicated<br>PRK – LASIK<br>LASIK<br>Non-corneal surgery | Glasses or CL |
| Hypermetropia | 0.00 to +1.50<br>+1.75 to +4.00<br>> +4.00 | Not indicated<br>PRK – LASIK<br>Not indicated | Glasses or CL |
| Astigmatism | 0.00 a 4.00<br>4.25 a 8.00<br>> 8.00 | PRK – LASIK<br>LASIK – Full arc incision<br>Not indicated | Glasses or CL |

All candidates for surgery must be informed of the expected results for their ametropy and the possible alternatives for correction, as well as the most frequent side effects and complications associated with the type of surgical procedure proposed[54].

# References

[1] Azar, DT. Refractive Surgery. Appleton andLange. Stamford, Connecticut. 1997.

[2] Albertazzi R, Centurión V. La moderna cirugía refractiva. Buenos Aires 1999.

[3] Talamo JH, Krueger RR. The excimer manual. A clinician's guide to excimer laser surgery. 1est Edition. Editorial Little, Brown and Company; 1997.

[4] Koch DD, Kohnen T, Obstbaum SA, Rosen ES. Format for reporting refractive surgical data. *J. Cataract. Refract. Surg.*. 1998;24:285-287.

[5] Martín R., Cirugía Refractiva y Optometría. Gaceta Óptica. 2001;350:10-15.

[6] Daya S. Refractive Surgery and Optometrist. www.optometry.co.uk 2000; 1:26-31.

[7] Duffey RJ, Leaming D. US trends in refractive surgery: 2003 ISRS/AAO survey. *J. Refract. Surg.* 2005;21:87-91.

[8] Barraquer JI. Cirugía refractiva de la córnea. Tomo I y II. Instituto Barraquer de América. Bogotá 1989.

[9] Waring GO, Lynn MJ, Mc Donnell PJ. Results of the prospective evaluation of radial keratotomy (PERK) study 10 years after surgery. *Arch. Ophthalmol.* 1994;112:1298-1308.

[10] Akura J, Matsuura K, Hatta S, Otsuka K, Kaneda S. A new concept for the correction of astigmatism: full-arc, depth-dependent astigmatic keratotomy. *Ophthalmology.* 2000;107:95-104.

[11] Güell JL, Vazquez M. Correction of high astigmatism with astigmatic keratotomy combined with laser in situ keratomileusis. *J. Cataract. Refract. Surg.* 2000;26:960-6.

[12] Stein HA, Cheskes A, Stein RM. The Excimer. Fundamentals and Clinical Use. Slack Incorporated 1995.

[13] Jimenez Alfaro I, Pérez Santonja JJ, Yáñez Mártinez J, Zato Gómez de Liaño M. Cirugía Refractiva con láser excímer. Tecnimedia Editorial 1995.

[14] Trokel SL, Srinivasan R, Braren B. Excimer laser surgery of the cornea. *Am. J. Ophthalmol.* 1983;96:710-715.

[15] www.fda.gov.

[16] Pallikaris IG, Kalyvianaki MI, Katsanevaki VJ, Ginis HS. Epi-LASIK: preliminary clinical results of an alternative surface ablation procedure. *J. Cataract. Refract. Surg.* 2005;31:879-85.

[17] Katsanevaki VJ, Kalyvianaki MI, Kavroulaki DS, Pallikaris IG. One-year clinical results after epi-LASIK for myopia. *Ophthalmology.* 2007;114:1111-7.

[18] Autrata R, Rehurek J. Laser-assisted subepithelial keratectomy for myopia: two-year follow-up. *J. Cataract. Refract Surg.* 2003;29:661-8.

[19] Hashemi H, Fotouhi A, Foudazi H, Sadeghi N, Payvar S. Prospective, randomized, paired comparison of laser epithelial keratomileusis and photorefractive keratectomy for myopia less than -6.50 diopters. *J. Refract Surg.* 2004;20:217-22.

[20] Ghirlando A, Gambato C, Midena E. LASEK and photorefractive keratectomy for myopia: clinical and confocal microscopy comparison. J Refract Surg. 2007;23:694-702.

[21] De Benito-Llopis L, Teus MA, Sánchez-Pina JM, Hernández-Verdejo JL. Comparison between LASEK and LASIK for the correction of low myopia. *J. Refract. Surg.* 2007;23:139-45.

[22] Teus MA, de Benito-Llopis L, Sánchez-Pina JM. LASEK versus LASIK for the correction of moderate myopia. *Optom Vis Sci.* 2007;84:605-10.

[23] O'Brart DP, Mellington F, Jones S, Marshall J. Laser epithelial keratomileusis for the correction of hyperopia using a 7.0-mm optical zone with the Schwind ESIRIS laser. *J. Refract. Surg.* 2007;23:343-54.

[24] McDonald MB, Beuerman R, Falzoni W, Rivera L, Kaufman HE. Refractive surgery with the excimer laser. *Am. J. Ophthalmo*l. 1987;15:103-469.

[25] McDonald MB, Frantz JM, Klyce SD, et al. One-year refractive results of central photorefractive keratectomy for myopia in the nonhuman primate cornea. *Arch. Ophthalmol.* 1990;108:40-7.

[26] Pallikaris IG, Papatzanaki ME, Stathi EZ, et al. Laser in situ keratomileusis. *Lasers Surg Med.* 1990;10:463-8.

[27] Pallikaris IG, Papatzanaki ME, Siganos DS, Tsilimbaris MK. A corneal flap technique for laser in situ keratomileusis. Human studies. *Arch. Ophthalmol.* 1991;109:1699-702.

[28] Pallikaris IG, Siganos DS. Excimer laser in situ keratomileusis and photorefractive keratectomy for correction of high myopia. *J. Refract Corneal Surg.* 1994;10:498-510.

[29] Güell JL, Arias A, Díez-Feijoó E. Queratomileusis in situ con laser excimer (LASIK) Sociedad Española de Oftalmología - Tecnimedia Editorial SL. España 1997.

[30] El-Maghraby A, Salah T, Waring GO 3rd, Klyce S, Ibrahim O. Randomized bilateral comparison of excimer laser in situ keratomileusis and photorefractive keratectomy for 2.50 to 8.00 diopters of myopia. *Ophthalmology.* 1999;106:447-57.

[31] Halkiadakis I, Belfair N, Gimbel H. Laser in situ keratomileusis in patients with diabetes. *J. Cataract Refract Surg.* 2005;31:1895–1898.

[32] Kim JY, Kim MJ, Kim TI, et al. A femtosecond laser creates a stronger flap than a mechanical microkeratome. *Invest Ophthalmol Vis Sci.* 2006;47:599-604.

[33] Lim T, Yang S, Kim M, Tchah H. Comparison of the IntraLase femtosecond laser and mechanical microkeratome for laser in situ keratomileusis. *Am J Ophthalmol.* 2006;141:833-9.

[34] Kezirian GM, Stonecipher KG. Comparison of the IntraLase femtosecond laser and mechanical keratomes for laser in situ keratomileusis. *J. Cataract Refract Surg.* 2004;30:804-11.

[35] Reviglio VE, Bossana EL, Luna JD, Muiño JC, Juarez CP. Laser in situ keratomileusis for myopia and hyperopia using the Lasersight 200 laser in 300 consecutive eyes. *J. Refract Surg.* 2000;16:716-23.

[36] Kermani O, Schmeidt K, Oberheide U, Gerten G. Hyperopic laser in situ keratomileusis with 5.5-, 6.5-, and 7.0-mm optical zones. *J. Refract Surg.* 2005;21:52-8.

[37] Ismail MM. LASIK using the NIDEK EC-5000 for the correction of hyperopic astigmatism. *J. Refract Surg.* 2006;22:1069-72.

[38] Choi RY, Wilson SE. Hyperopic laser in situ keratomileusis: primary and secondary treatments are safe and effective. *Cornea*. 2001;20:388-93.

[39] Randleman JB, Lynn MJ, Banning CS, Stulting RD. Risk factors for epithelial defect formation during laser in situ keratomileusis. *J. Cataract Refract Surg*. 2007;33:1738-43.

[40] Landau D, Levy J, Solomon A, et al. Traumatic corneal flap dislocation one to six years after LASIK in nine eyes with a favorable outcome. *J. Refract Surg*. 2006;22:884-9.

[41] Ramírez M, Quiroz-Mercado H, Hernandez-Quintela E, Naranjo-Tackman R. Traumatic flap dislocation 4 years after LASIK due to air bag injury. *J. Refract Surg*. 2007;23:729-30.

[42] Pereira Cda R, Narvaez J, King JA, Seery LS, Gimbel HV. Late-onset traumatic dislocation with central tissue loss of laser in situ keratomileusis flap. *Cornea*. 2006;25:1107-10.

[43] Nilforoushan MR, Speaker MG, Latkany R. Traumatic flap dislocation 4 years after laser in situ keratomileusis. *J. Cataract Refract Surg*. 2005;31:1664-5.

[44] Tahzib N, Bootsma S, Eggink F, Nabar V, Nuijts R. Functional outcomes and patient satisfaction after laser in situ keratomileusis for correction of myopia. *J. Cataract Refract Surg*. 2005;31:1943–1951.

[45] Lin RT, Maloney RK. Flap complications associated with lamellar refractive surgery. *Am J Ophthalmol*. 1999;127:129-36.

[46] Gimbel HV, Penno EE, van Westenbrugge JA, et al. Incidence and management of intraoperative and early postoperative complications in 1000 consecutive laser in situ keratomileusis cases. *Ophthalmology*. 1998;105:1839-47.

[47] Stulting RD, Carr JD, Thompson KP, et al. Complications of laser in situ keratomileusis for the correction of myopia. *Ophthalmology*. 1999;106:13-20.

[48] Cheng AC, Wong VW, Rao SK, Lam DS. Repositioning of free cap four days after LASIK. *J. Refract Surg*. 2007;23:625-7.

[49] Kymionis GD, Diakonis VF, Bouzoukis DI, et al. Idiopathic recurrence of diffuse lamellar keratitis after LASIK. *J. Refract Surg*. 2007;23:720-1.

[50] Walker MB, Wilson SE. Incidence and prevention of epithelial growth within the interface after laser in situ keratomileusis. *Cornea*. 2000;19:170-3.

[51] Sun L, Liu G, Ren Y, et al. Efficacy and safety of LASIK in 10,052 eyes of 5081 myopic Chinese patients. *J. Refract Surg*. 2005;21:S633-5.

[52] Mackool RJ, Monsanto VR. Epithelial ingrowth after LASIK. *J. Cataract Refract Surg*. 2002;28:1884.

[53] Randleman JB, Banning CS, Stulting RD. Persistent epithelial ingrowth. *Ophthalmology*. 2006;113:1468.

[54] Fong CS. Refractive surgery: the future of perfect vision?. Singapore *Med J*. 2007;48:709-18.

[55] Lichter H, Stulting RD, Waring GO 3rd, Russell GE, Carr J. Buttonholes during LASIK: etiology and outcome. *J. Refract Surg*. 2007;23:472-6.

[56] Tuisku IS, Lindbohm N, Wilson SE, Tervo TM. Dry eye and corneal sensitivity after high myopic LASIK. *J. Refract. Surg*. 2007;23:338-42.

[57] Shoja MR, Besharati MR. Dry eye after LASIK for myopia: Incidence and risk factors. Eur J Ophthalmol. 2007;17:1-6.

[58] Chan CC, Boxer Wachler BS. Comparison of the effects of LASIK retreatment techniques on epithelial ingrowth rates. *Ophthalmology*. 2007;114:640-2.

[59] Marcos S, Barbero S, Llorente L, Merayo-Lloves J. Optical response to LASIK surgery for myopia from total and corneal aberration measurements. *Invest. Ophthalmol. Vis. Sci.* 2001;42:3349-56.

[60] Llorente L, Barbero S, Merayo J, Marcos S. Total and corneal optical aberrations induced by laser in situ keratomileusis for hyperopia. *J. Refract Surg.* 2004;20:203-16.

[61] Marcos S. Aberrations and visual performance following standard laser vision correction. *J. Refract Surg.* 2001;17:596-601.

[62] Oshika T, Klyce SD, Applegate RA, Howland HC, El Danasoury MA. Comparison of corneal wavefront aberrations after photorefractive keratectomy and laser in situ keratomileusis. *Am J Ophthalmol.* 1999;127:1-7.

[63] Jabbur NS, Stark WJ, Green WR. Corneal ectasia after laser-assisted in situ keratomileusis. *Arch Ophthalmol.* 2001;119:1714-6.

[64] Piccoli PM, Gomes AA, Piccoli FV. Corneal ectasia detected 32 months after LASIK for correction of myopia and asymmetric astigmatism. *J. Cataract Refract Surg.* 2003;29:1222-5.

[65] Kanellopoulos AJ. Post-LASIK ectasia. *Ophthalmology*. 2007;114:1230.

[66] Condon PI, O'Keefe M, Binder PS. Long-term results of laser in situ keratomileusis for high myopia: risk for ectasia. *J. Cataract. Refract. Surg.* 2007;33:583-90.

[67] Panagopoulou SI, Pallikaris IG. Wavefront customized ablations with the WASCA Asclepion workstation. *J. Refract Surg.* 2001;17:S608-12.

[68] Kanjani N, Jacob S, Agarwal A, et al. Wavefront- and topography-guided ablation in myopic eyes using Zyoptix. *J. Cataract Refract Surg.* 2004;30:285-6.

[69] Mastropasqua L, Nubile M, Ciancaglini M, Toto L, Ballone E. Prospective randomized comparison of wavefront-guided and conventional photorefractive keratectomy for myopia with the meditec MEL 70 laser. *J. Refract Surg.* 2004;20:422-31.

[70] Kim TI, Yang SJ, Tchah H. Bilateral comparison of wavefront-guided versus conventional laser in situ keratomileusis with Bausch and Lomb Zyoptix. *J. Refract Surg.* 2004;20:432-8.

[71] Tran DB, Sarayba MA, Bor Z, Garufis C, Duh YJ, Soltes CR, Juhasz T, Kurtz RM. Randomized prospective clinical study comparing induced aberrations with IntraLase and Hansatome flap creation in fellow eyes: potential impact on wavefront-guided laser in situ keratomileusis. *J. Cataract Refract Surg.* 2005;31:97-105.

[72] Patel SV, Maguire LJ, McLaren JW, Hodge DO, Bourne WM. Femtosecond laser versus mechanical microkeratome for LASIK: a randomized controlled study. *Ophthalmology*. 2007;114:1482-90.

[73] Venter J. Wavefront-guided LASIK with the NIDEK NAVEX platform for the correction of myopia and myopic astigmatism with 6-month follow-up. *J. Refract Surg* 2005;21:S640-5.

[74] Caster AI, Hoff JL, Ruiz R. Conventional vs wavefront-guided LASIK using the LADARVision4000 excimer laser. *J. Refract Surg.* 2005;21:S786-91.

[75] Awwad ST, Haithcock KK, Oral D, et al. A comparison of induced astigmatism in conventional and wavefront-guided myopic LASIK using LADARVision4000 and VISX S4 platforms. *J. Refract Surg.* 2005;21:S792-8.
[76] Bahar I, Levinger S, Kremer I. Wavefront-guided LASIK for myopia with the Technolas 217Z: results at 3 years. *J. Refract. Surg.* 2007;23:586-90.
[77] Binder PS. Analysis of ectasia after laser in situ keratomileusis: risk factors. *J. Cataract Refract Surg.* 2007;33:1530-8.
[78] Randleman JB, Russell B, Ward MA, Thompson KP, Stulting RD. Risk factors and prognosis for corneal ectasia after LASIK. *Ophthalmology.* 2003;110:267-75.
[79] Klein SR, Epstein RJ, Randleman JB, Stulting RD. Corneal ectasia after laser in situ keratomileusis in patients without apparent preoperative risk factors. *Cornea.* 2006;25:388-403.
[80] McDonald MB. Conductive keratoplasty: a radiofrequency-based technique for the correction of hyperopia. *Trans Am Ophthalmol Soc.* 2005;103:512-36.
[81] McDonald MB, Hersh PS, Manche EE, et al. Conductive keratoplasty for the correction of low to moderate hyperopia: U.S. clinical trial 1-year results on 355 eyes. *Ophthalmology.* 2002;109:1978-89.
[82] Summary of Safety and Effectiveness Data ViewPoint CK System Refractec. FDA web. 2002 (http://www.fda.gov).
[83] Du TT, Fan VC, Asbell PA. Conductive keratoplasty. *Curr Opin Ophthalmol.* 2007;18:334-7.
[84] Rocha G, Castillo JM, Sanchez-Thorin JC, et al. Two-year follow-up of noncontact holmium laser thermokeratoplasty for the correction of low hyperopia. *Can J Ophthalmol.* 2003;38:385-92.
[85] J.L Menezo; J.L. Güell Corrección Quirúrgica de la Alta Miopía. Ed. Espaxs SA Barcelona 2001.
[86] Jiménez-Alfaro I, Miguelez S, Bueno JL, Puy P. Clear lens extraction and implantation of negative-power posterior chamber intraocular lenses to correct extreme myopia. *J. Cataract Refract Surg* .1998;24:1310-1316.
[87] Colin J, Robinet A, Cochener B. Retinal detachment after clear lens extraction for high myopia: seven-years follow-up. *Ophthalmology* 1999;106: 2281-4.
[88] Martínez-Castillo V, Boixadera A, Verdugo A, et al. Rhegmatogenous retinal detachment in phakic eyes after posterior chamber phakic intraocular lens implantation for severe myopia. *Ophthalmology.* 2005;112:580-5.
[89] Arne JL. Phakic intraocular lens implantation versus clear lens extraction in highly myopic eyes of 30- to 50-year-old patients. *J. Cataract Refract Surg.* 2004;30:2092-6.
[90] Fernández-Vega L, Alfonso JF, Villacampa T. Clear lens extraction for the correction of high myopia. *Ophthalmology.* 2003;110:2349-54.
[91] Fernández-Vega L, Alfonso JF, Rodríguez PP, Montés-Micó R. Clear lens extraction with multifocal apodized diffractive intraocular lens implantation. *Ophthalmology.* 2007;114:1491-8.
[92] Pérez-Santonja JJ, Bueno JL, Zato MA. Surgical correction of high myopia in phakic eyes with Worst-Fechner myopia intraocular lenses. *J. Refract. Surg* .1997;13:268-284.

[93] Coullet J, Guëll JL, Fournié P, et al. Iris-supported phakic lenses (rigid vs foldable version) for treating moderately high myopia: randomized paired eye comparison. *Am. J. Ophthalmol.* 2006;142:909-16.

[94] Moshirfar M, Holz HA, Davis DK. Two-year follow-up of the Artisan/Verisyse iris-supported phakic intraocular lens for the correction of high myopia. *J. Cataract Refract Surg.* 2007;33:1392-7.

[95] Benedetti S, Casamenti V, Benedetti M. Long-term endothelial changes in phakic eyes after Artisan intraocular lens implantation to correct myopia: five-year study. *J. Cataract Refract Surg.* 2007;33:784-90.

[96] Bootsma SJ, Tahzib NG, Eggink FA, et al. Evaluation of pupil dynamics after implantation of artisan phakic intraocular lenses. *J. Refract Surg.* 2006;22:367-71.

[97] Sanders D, Vukich JA. Comparison of implantable collamer lens (ICL) and laser-assisted in situ keratomileusis (LASIK) for low myopia. *Cornea.* 2006;25:1139-46.

[98] Sanders DR. Matched population comparison of the Visian Implantable Collamer Lens and standard LASIK for myopia of -3.00 to -7.88 diopters. *J. Refract Surg.* 2007;23:537-53.

[99] Sanders DR, Schneider D, Martin R, et al. Toric Implantable Collamer Lens for moderate to high myopic astigmatism. *Ophthalmology.* 2007;114:54-61.

[100] Sanders DR, Doney K, Poco M, et al. United States Food and Drug Administration clinical trial of the Implantable Collamer Lens (ICL) for moderate to high myopia: three-year follow-up. *Ophthalmology.* 2004;111:1683-92.

[101] Shipper I. Surgical management of acute angle-closure glaucoma after implantation of a toric ICL. *J. Cataract Refract Surg.* 2007;33:563-4.

[102] Zaldivar R, Oscherow S, Piezzi V. Bioptics in phakic and pseudophakic intraocular lens with the Nidek EC-5000 excimer laser. *J. Refract Surg.* 2002;18:S336-9.

[103] Alfonso JF, Fernández-Vega L, Señaris A, Montés-Micó R. Quality of vision with the Acri.Twin asymmetric diffractive bifocal intraocular lens system. *J. Cataract Refract Surg.* 2007;33:197-202.

[104] Chiam PJ, Chan JH, Aggarwal RK, Kasaby S. ReSTOR intraocular lens implantation in cataract surgery: quality of vision. *J. Cataract Refract Surg.* 2006;32:1459-63.

[105] Artigas JM, Menezo JL, Peris C, Felipe A, Díaz-Llopis M. Image quality with multifocal intraocular lenses and the effect of pupil size: comparison of refractive and hybrid refractive-diffractive designs. *J. Cataract Refract Surg.* 2007;33:2111-7.

[106] Mester U, Hunold W, Wesendahl T, Kaymak H. Functional outcomes after implantation of Tecnis ZM900 and Array SA40 multifocal intraocular lenses. *J. Cataract Refract Surg.* 2007;33:1033-40.

[107] Alfonso JF, Fernández-Vega L, Baamonde MB, Montés-Micó R. Prospective visual evaluation of apodized diffractive intraocular lenses. *J. Cataract Refract Surg.* 2007;33:1235-43.

[108] Souza CE, Muccioli C, Soriano ES, Chalita MR, et al. Visual performance of AcrySof ReSTOR apodized diffractive IOL: a prospective comparative trial. *Am J. Ophthalmol.* 2006;141:827-832.

[109] Vingolo EM, Grenga P, Iacobelli L, Grenga R. Visual acuity and contrast sensitivity: AcrySof ReSTOR apodized diffractive versus AcrySof SA60AT monofocal intraocular lenses. *J. Cataract Refract Surg.* 2007;33:1244-7.

[110] Sen HN, Sarikkola AU, Uusitalo RJ, Laatikainen L. Quality of vision after AMO Array multifocal intraocular lens implantation. *J. Cataract Refract Surg.* 2004;30:2483-93.

[111] Pepose JS, Qazi MA, Davies J, Doane JF, Loden JC, Sivalingham V, Mahmoud AM. Visual performance of patients with bilateral vs combination Crystalens, ReZoom, and ReSTOR intraocular lens implants. *Am J. Ophthalmol.* 2007;144:347-357.

[112] Salati C, Salvetat ML, Zeppieri M, Brusini P. Pupil size influence on the intraocular performance of the multifocal AMO-Array intraocular lens in elderly patients. *Eur J. Ophthalmol.* 2007;17:571-8.

[113] Elgohary M, Zaheer A, Werner L, Ionides A, Sheldrick J, Ahmed N. Opacification of Array SA40N silicone multifocal intraocular lens. *J. Cataract Refract Surg.* 2007;33:342-7.

In: Laser Keratectomy: Approaches, Complications...
Author: Luis W. Schröder and Felix J. Walter
ISBN 978-1-60456-863-9


*Chapter III*

# Refractive Surgery and Infections

***Antonio M.Fea, Valeria Guglielmi, Alessandro G.Actis, and Federico M. Grignolo***
Department of Clinical Physiopathology, Ophthalmology Section, Turin University, Italy

## Abstract

*Introduction:* Infections are potentially devastating in ocular surgery and several reviews and multicenter trials have been dealing with infection following cataract surgery. Both in LASIK and in PRK infections might have a serious course and determine poor refractive results and in some cases lead to keratoplasty.

*Matherial and methods:* a meta-analysis of the literature was performed. PRK and LASIK were considered separately.

*Results*: Infections following refractive surgery (both PRK and LASIK) are extremely rare. The great majority of infections were caused by gram positive bacteria. Preferred therapy is by fourth generation fluoroquinolones. There is no accepted prevention of the infection in the literature. When comparing the occurrence of infections in PRK and LASIK similar prevalence was found.

*Conclusions:* Although rare, infections following refractive surgery are potentially devastating. Accurate prevention of infection is described in this review. Most of the infections occur during the first week and accurate follow up is recommended during the first few days following the procedure. Identification of the infective agent is important in order to start a targeted therapy.

## Lasik

In November 2001 [1] the ASCRS (The American Society of Cataract and Refractive Surgery) Cornea Clinical Committee conducted one of the principal studies on post-LASIK infections, sending an e-mail with a questionnaire to 8600 American and International members to assess the incidence of infectious keratitises after LASIK, with case samples of 338,550 eyes and 56 surgeons.

The septic keratitises identified were 116 cases subdivided as follows:

- staphylococci: 23
- atypical mycobacteria : 33
- others: 13
- negative culture: 26
- no culture: 21

It is interesting to note that the use of the Lowenstein-Jensen medium on which the Nocardia (atypical mycobacteria) grows, becuase it is the most common organism seen after Lasik. The therapy should be chosen according to the clinical characterization of the keratitis:

- rapid onset keratitis: fluoroquinolones + vancomicyn 50mg/ml every 30 minutes+doxycycline 100mg twice daily and corticosteroids periodically
- -delayed-onset keratitis: (e.g.:Nocardia atypical mycobacteria and fungi) amikacin 20 mg/ml per day every 30 minutes alternated with vancomicyn 50mg/ml every 30 minutes, doxycycline 100mg twice daily and corticosteroids periodically, alternatively clarithromycin and fourth generation fluoroquinolones can also be used.

Empirical therapy is never recommended because many organisms are opportunist and do not respond to such therapy.

Chang in a 2004 meta-analysis [2] assessed 103 infections in 87 patients (extracted from 42 articles) of which 74.7% patients were operated on by other surgeons.

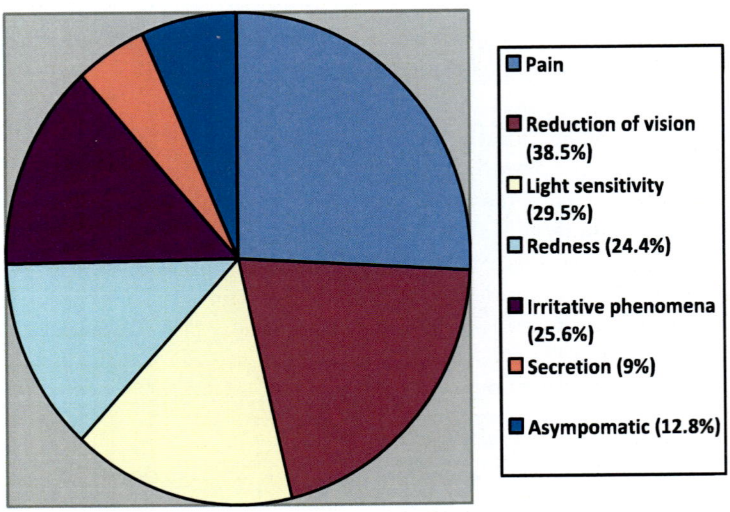


Graphic 1. symptoms in Chang Metanalisis.

**Table 1.Microbiological profile in Chang metanalisis**

| Time of organism identification | Total number of eyes | Microbiological agent | Number of Keratoplasties | Mean Snellen AV media |
|---|---|---|---|---|
| = or < 7 gg | 28 | 23 Gram+<br>5 Mycobatterium<br>1 Fungal<br>1 Pseudomonas | 7 | 20/37 |
| > 7 gg | 44 | 25 Mycobatterium<br>8 Fungus<br>5 Yeast<br>3 Polymicrobial<br>2 Gram +<br>1 Acanthamoeba | 7 | 20/83 |

Significant differences by gender or eye were not observed. 87% of infections appeared after the first operation, 13% after re-operation. The data were stratified according to pathogenic agent, type of post-operative treatment, visual decline. No risk factor was identified, 15 patients out of 16 with bilateral infection underwent a bilateral procedure, the information on post-operative antibiotics was collected for 39 patients (with 16 using fluoroquinolones and 14 tobramycin). Information on specific symptoms was available on 78 eyes (Graphic 1).

Only 6.3% invaded both the stroma and the flap. Ulcers represent 11.7%, abscesses 3.9%, reaction in AC 23.3%, and new epithelial defects 35.9%.

Gram + bacteria are usually associated with pain, secretion, epithelial deficit, reaction in the anterior chamber, separation of the flap. Fungi are usually associated with conjunctival hyperemia, lacrimation. Mycobacteria do not have particular associations.

Information on the onset and the frequency of infections was available for 83 eyes, 41 were infected in less than a week with an average time of 2.7 days, principally by gram+, while 42 eyes after 10 days with average time of 27.4 days, principally by mycobacteria.

A microbiological profile was performed on 72 eyes evaluating the time for the identification of the microrganism, the possible need for corneal transplant and the final Snellen visual acuity average (see table 1)

The conclusions of this broad meta-analysis lead us to report that infection frequency is very variable, despite the prophylaxis (Fluoroquinolones), infections have occurred (only Gram -), no predisposing factor could be identified. When operating bilaterally a greater frequency of infection is possible which may also lead to serious visual deficit. 21 cases were mistaken for DLK and treated with steroids initially, indeed at times symptomology is insufficient to allow diagnosis and the infiltrates may present even without epithelial damage.

# Differential Diagnosis

Differential diagnosis is possible with:
Non-septic opacities of the interface which present:

- epithelial cells
- metallic microfragments (microkeratome)
- powders

## DLK

- The infiltrate of DLK has specific clinical characteristics:
- It is an infiltrate with well defined boarders
- It is limited in extension to the interface
- It is characterised as a linear white granular interface infiltrate pattern, resembling the shifting desert sands

The inflammation process in the anterior chamber is limited in extent or absent
There is no overlying of epithelial defect

## Prk Vs Lasik:

De Oliveira et al [3] compared the two surgical techniques in terms of effectiveness and of risk of infiltrates (infectious or inflammatory). Of the 8,508 eyes examined (Refractive Surgery Outpatient Clinic-Vision Institute in San Paulo) during the 60 days post-operative period, 4492 were treated with PRK and 4016 with Lasik. Cases with infiltrates with infectious or inflammatory characteristics were included, while cases with a probable viral etiology unrelated to surgery (multiple and subepithelial infiltrates without edema) and those with the characteristics of DLK were excluded. Of the 4492 PRK eyes, 35 were positive and of the 4016 LASIK ones, only 4 were positive, with an incidence of 0.8% , compared to 0.1% in LASIK. A greater incidence of infections in PRK has been attributed to the surgical technique; in fact the former technique produces 6 to 8 mm epithelial defect, which takes approximately 4 days to heal. In addition in PRK therapeutic contact lenses are used for 4 days after the operation to reduce pain and to accelerate the corneal re-epithelialisation, but they mightincrease the risk of infection (see PRK below). The time of diagnosis post-PRK varies between 3 and 21 days with an average of 6 days, while for LASIK it is between 1 and 6 days with an average of 4 days. The infiltrates found were always monolateral. This fact owes very probably to the choice of the surgeon to wait one week before the fellow eye procedure, in order to avoid bilateral infections and to assess the visual result. At the end of every operation tobramycin and dexamethasone were applied. Corneal scraping was done for all the 16 infiltrates whith clinical characteristics of an inflammatory process underway, 10 of these were positive for Gram + bacterial infections. 9 were PRK-tretaed eyes and 1 LASIK-treated eye. (see table 2). For the LASIK treated eye, the positive culture infiltrate was located at the superior temporal flap edge. Of the 9 eyes treated by PRK, the locations of the positive culture infiltrates included the superior (n=1), inferior (n=2), nasal superior (n=1), central (n=2) and nasal inferior (n=2) regions of the cornea.

**Table 2. Bacterial infections in De Oliveira study**

| BACTERIA | NUMBER OF POSITIVE CULTURES |
|---|---|
| Corinebacterium xerosis | 1 |
| Streptococcus viridans | 1 |
| Staphylococcus aureus | 2 |
| Coagulase-negative Staphylococcus | 5 |
| Gram-positive coccus | 1 |

Of the eyes infected, 14 were treated with cefazolin and gentamicin, 1 with cefazolin and 1 with oflaxicin and vancomicyn.

The resolution time of the infiltrate varied between 1 day and 1 month with an average of 10 days.

All the authors recommend an appropriate conjunctival culture.

The bacteria most frequently detected post-operatively were the Gram-positive cocci, while on the pre-operative strip they were coagulase-negative Staphylococci.

In 95% of the cases post-operative visual acuity was greater or equal to 8/10.

## PRK

Wroblewski et al [4] analysed the keratitis after PRK data taken from 6 Army and Navy refractive surgery centers with a total of 25,337 PRK performed in 6 centres between January 1995 and May 2004. All patients received prophylaxis with antibiotic eyedrops pre-operatively. Five keratitis were reported in five different patients in the first week post-operatively: four were caused by methicillin resistant Staphylococcus Aureus (MRSA), 1 case was only a presumed keratitis, negative to the culture.

The data of these 5 patients are resumed in table 3.

**Table 3. patients data in Wroblewski study**

| Day of presentation | Antibiotic post-surgery | Culture | F-U (mos) | Final UCVA |
|---|---|---|---|---|
| 6 | Ofloxacin | MRSA | 5 | 0,67 |
| 2 | Politrim | Staphylococcus Aureus | 3 | 0,8 |
| 3 | Levofloxacin | MRSA | 7 | 1,2 |
| 7 | Ofloxacin | Negative | 12 | 1 |
| 3 | Ofloxacin | Coaugulase-Staphylococcus | 12 | 1 |

(F-U: follow-up; MRSA: methicillin-resistant Staphylococcus avaible; UCVA uncorrected visual acuity)

Here we analyze the individual cases:

CASE 1: The patient was operated for myopia and astigmatism. On the 4th post-operatively day the patient presented a minimal epithelial defect in both eyes and the BCLs were changed. On the sixth day there was a worsening of the symptomology with redness and pain. The objective test revealed a partial corneal infiltrate with cells in the AC and hypopion. The BCL is removed and a culture was performed. The ofloxacin begun immediately after the operation was interrupted and replaced by fortified topical antibiotics such as vancomicyn and gentamicin. On the tenth day post-operatively the culture was positive for the methicillin resistant Staphylococcus (MRSA). Gentamicin was interrupted, the patient continues with Vancomicyn every hour. Patient treated with mupirocin calcium. After 21 days the infiltrate was resolved and the epithelium healed with central haze and at the end VA of 0.6.

CASE 2: PRK in both the eyes. The first day post-operatively manifested a VA of 0.6. On the second day post-operatively he began to rub the eye and to manifest pain with a considerable reduction of the VA ad 0.1 with a reduced epithelial defect central a level corneal without infiltrates. On the fourth day post-operatively LAC was absent, the epithelial defect had increased, the corneal infiltrates were multiple, there were keratic precipitates and hypopion. The attack therapy on the fourth day post-operatively was Cefazolin + modified Tobramycin replacing the Tobramycin with Ciproflaxicin on the sixth day post-operatively for St Aureus culture positivity. After a month the corneal epithelium appeared healed with a residual haze and UCVA after three months was of 0.8 (Figure1).

CASE 3: Operated on with PRK in both the eyes for myopia and astigmatism. On the first day post operatively the UCVAs was of 0,6. The third day post-operatively presented an increase in the pain and a reduction of visual acuity and conjunctival redness with a VA of (20/160) and a central epithelial infiltrate BCL was removed and a culture was performed. Fortified antibiotics such as cefazolin and gentamicin started. The culture tested positive for MRSA and the antibiotics were replaced by vancomicyn. Three months later VA was of (20/16) with a central corneal haze. After 6 months the VA was of 20/16.

CASE 4: Patient operated on for hyperopia. On the VI day post-operatively the patient manifested an epithelial defect of 1-2 mm, and LAC was changed, on the VII day the epithelium appears reformed, but there is stromal infiltrate. LAC was removed, the Oflaxicin was increased every hour and the cefazolin and eritromicina were dripped 4 times per day. On the VIII day the first infiltrate was being resolved, but there is the appearance of a new infiltrate, the cultures tested negative and the VA final was of 0.1.

CASE 5: Patient operated on for myopia and astigmatism. The III day post-operative presented a infiltrate with epithelial defect and reaction in AC. The culture tested positive for Staphylococcus coagulase negative. LAC was removed and the therapy formulated is Oflaxicin every hour with cefazolin and eritromicina. The VA at the end was of 0.1 (Figure2).

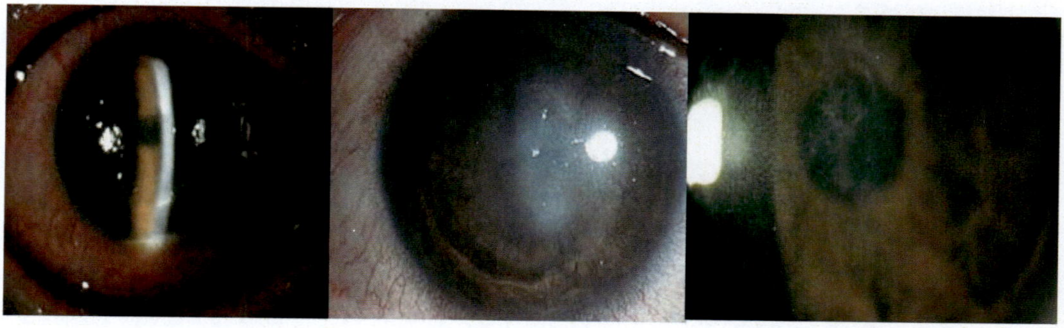

Figure 1.

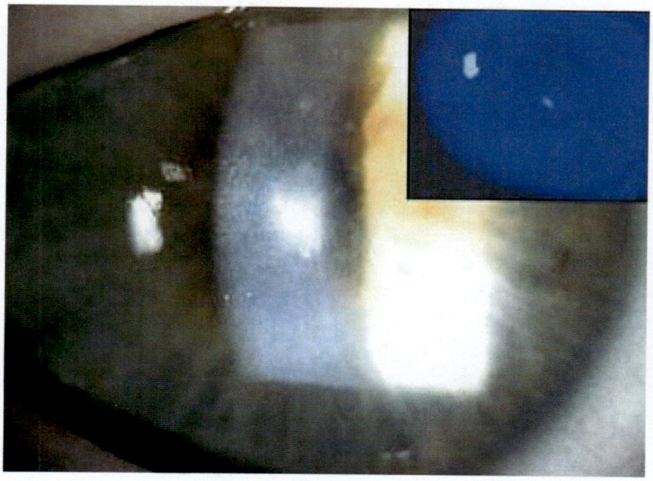

Figure 2.

A further 26 eyes considered sterile developed corneal infiltrates in the first week post-operatively. In three of these the cultures were negative with infiltrates for the more peripheral ones with dimensions equal to or less than 2 mm and epithelium intact or punctate epitheliopathy. Some developed the infection outside the area treated surgically. All were treated with success with removal of the LAC and with a increase of the topical antibiotic therapy (fluoroquinolones) and giving gram + protection (bacitracin or erithromycin). Only one patient had a VA reduced by 1 line.

Pre and post-operative antibiotics are useful as prophylaxis even if the rate of incidence of infections is low.

The presentation of corneal infiltrates in the first postoperative week after PRK necessitates aggressive treatment. Post operative infections manifest themselves in most cases in the first week.

# PRK and Rare Infections

Kouyoumdjian et al [5] analysed a rare case of infection of a patient in a 36 years old patient who underwent bilateral PRK. After LAC removal the patient began to complain of pain and sight reduction

The objective test revealed a central infiltrate and visual acuity was reduced to hand motion. The therapy was Oflaxicin every 2 h; Prednisolone x 4

After 3 weeks was isolated the microorganism Scopulariopsis.

Despite intensive treatment PK (penetrating keratoplasty) remains the only possible solution (Figure3).

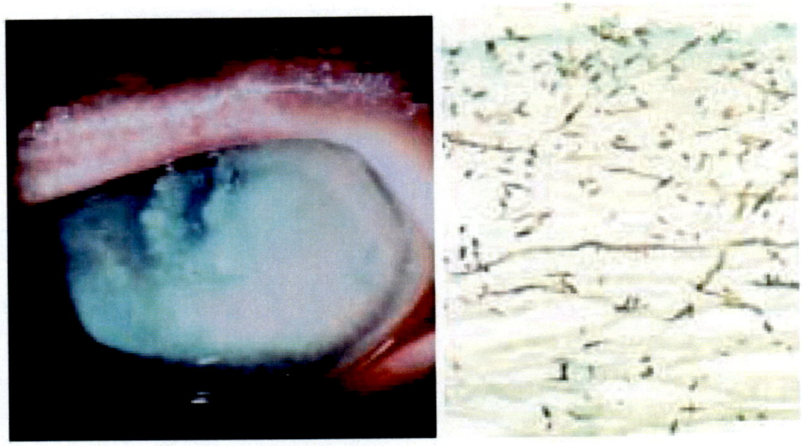

Figure 3.

Moshirfar et al [6] reported the first two cases of bacterial keratitis resistant to fourth generation fluoroquinolones after treatment with LASIK and with PRK. The fluoroquinolones are commonly used as prophylaxis for their broad spectrum of action against Gram+ and Gram- .

The first case was a myopic bilateral PRK patient with dry eye, who, one week after the operation, presented a muco-purulent corneal ulcer and subsequent hypopion, despite the antibiotics. The culture was positive for Pseudomonas aeruginosa. The therapy with was vancomicyn resolved the hypopion but not the central Descemetocele which led the patient to penetrating keratoplasty.

The second case was bilateral myopic LASIK patient. The first day post-operatively the patient presented pain and monolateral irritation. Corneal infiltrates were detected and therapy with Vigamox and Zymar was begun. VA was reduced and the pain continued to increase. After 17 days VA was hand motion, the cornea was edematose with epithelial defect and infiltrates and hypopion. A therapeutic contact lens was applied and the therapy was modified with vancomicyn and amikacin. Initial improvement with the new therapy was registered, but a central epithelial defect with moderate necrosis was still present after 5 days. Amputation of the necrotic central flap and continuation of the topical therapy for a further month resulted in a final VA of 0,3.

The fourth generation of fluoroquinolones has a good effect against the Staphylococcus aureus (MSSA) but a weak one against the methicillin resistant Staphylococcus aureus (MRSA) and against the pseudomonas aeruginosa.

It is important to recognise the limits of certain antibiotics. It is appropriate to treat post refractive surgery infections with associated antibiotics belonging to different classes. Factors causing the infections are dry eye (dry keratoconjunctivitis), anaesthetic and cortisonic eyedrops used for prolonged periods and the use of therapeutic contact lenses.

## LAC and PRK

Therapeutic contact lenses are used to reduce post-operative pain and to facilitate corneal re-epithelialization but they may increase the risk of microbial keratitis.

Detorakis et al [7], analyzed 60 lenses taken from 60 different eyes, established that 18.3% LAC (11 LAC) after PRK were colonised by Staphylococcus epidermidis, neither fungi nor other bacteria were found. Women were more affected and this has led to the presumption that cosmetics were a possible cause and the eyelids a possible source of infection.

Dantas [8] analyzed 81 eyes PRK treated. Immediately after each procedure, disposable soft contact lenses were positioned. After 3 days the lenses were removed. Seven positive culture were found: six gram positive cocci (7.4 %) and one gram negative bacillus (1.2%). There was no clinical correlation with these findings.

Hart et to the [9] considered 108 lenses taken from 41 patients (81 dailes and 26 non-dailies) and attempted to identify eventual pathogenic agents (bacterial, fungal). In 41 lenses pathogens were found. In 31 the pathogenic isolated agent was Staphylococcus epidermidis. The lenses which had been applied for a longer time were those with a greater number of colonies.

Radford [10] assessed the risk factors by means of a questionnaire of patients who presented themselves to the Moorfields Eye Hospital accident and Emergency Department with a diagnosis of microbial keratitis. The possible risk factors for microbial keratitis were the use of weekly lenses compared with dailies and the misuse of these in terms of hours.

Liesegang [11] has found that the incidence rates for bacterial microbial keratitis range from approximately two/10.000 per year for rigid contact lens, 2.2-4.1/10.000 per year for daily-wear soft contact lens, to 13.3-20.9/10.000 per year for extended-wear soft contact lenses. The risk with therapeutic contact lenses is much higher: approximately 52/10.000 per year. Amongst the most significant risk factors are overnight wear, smoking, male sex, and socioeconomic status. It is necessary to reduce the risk factors by means of clear communication with the patient.

Stern et al [12] have established a proneness to develop bacterial keratitis in contact lens wearers with a damaged corneal epithelium, poor care and hygiene of the lens, misuse of the same with consequent hypoxia. Soft lenses have the advantage of adapting well on the corneal surface, limiting deposits and the possibility of bacteria adhering and damage on greater oxygen flow.

# Conclusions

Infections after refractive surgery are infrequent, but potentially very dangerous.

Surgery is not always indispensable.

Refractive surgery is largely a non-essential procedure. Primary prevention in advisable, but secondary prevention of potentially serious corneal infections is essential to guarantee optimal refractive visual results. Patients should be informed of the symptoms and followed up strictly in the post-operative period when infections are more frequent. In the event of a suspect infection conjunctival culture should be performed to identify the causative agent and aggressive treatment should be given promptly.

# References


[1] Chang MA, Jain S, Azar DT. Infections following laser in situ keratomileusis: an integration of the published literature. *Surv. Ophthalmol.* 2004;49:269-80.

[2] de Oliveira GC, Solari HP, Ciola FB, et al. Corneal infiltrates after excimer laser photorefractive keratectomy and LASIK. *J. Refract. Surg.* 2006;22:159-65.

[3] Wroblewski KJ, Pasternak JF, Bower KS, et al. Infectious keratitis after photorefractive keratectomy in the United States army and navy. *Ophthalmology* 2006;113:520-5.

[4] Kouyoumdjian GA, Forstot SL, Durairaj VD, Damiano RE. Infectious keratitis after laser refractive surgery. *Ophthalmology* 2001;108:1266-8.

[5] Moshirfar M, Mirzaian G, Feiz V, Kang PC. Fourth-generation fluoroquinolone-resistant bacterial keratitis after refractive surgery. *J. Cataract. Refract. Surg.* 2006;32:515-8.

[6] Detorakis ET, Siganos DS, Houlakis VM, et al. Microbiological examination of bandage soft contact lenses used in laser refractive surgery. *J. Refract. Surg.* 1998;14:631-5.

[7] Dantas PE, Nishiwaki-Dantas MC, Ojeda VH, et al. Microbiological study of disposable soft contact lenses after photorefractive keratectomy. *CLAO J.* 2000;26:26-9.

[8] Hart DE, Reindel W, Proskin HM, Mowrey-McKee MF. Microbial contamination of hydrophilic contact lenses: quantitation and identification of microorganisms associated with contact lenses while on the eye. *Optom. Vis. Sci.* 1993;70:185-91.

[9] Radford CF, Minassian DC, Dart JK. Disposable contact lens use as a risk factor for microbial keratitis. *Br. J. Ophthalmol.* 1998;82:1272-5.

[10] Liesegang TJ. Contact lens-related microbial keratitis: Part I: Epidemiology. Cornea 1997;16:125-31.

[11] Stern GA. Contact lens associated bacterial keratitis: past, present, and future. *CLAO J.* 1998;24:52-6


We aknowledge the permission of using the photos taken from the articles quoted in the text by Elsevier.

In: Laser Keratectomy: Approaches, Complications... ISBN 978-1-60456-863-9
Author: Luis W. Schröder and Felix J. Walter


*Chapter IV*

# Lift-and-Scrape Technique for Laser-Assisted Subepithelial Keratectomy (LASEK)

***Raymond I. Cho*[1], *Ava Huchun*[2], *and Kraig S. Bower*[3*]**
[1]Department of Ophthalmology, University of Michigan; [2]Ophthalmology Service, Ft. Stewart, Georgia, [3]Walter Reed Army Medical Center, Washington, District of Columbia, USA

## Abstract

The alcohol-assisted manual technique used to lift the corneal epithelium during laser-assisted subepithelial keratectomy (LASEK) often results in stretching of the epithelial flap, causing the flap edges to overlap the border of peripheral epithelium. We describe a lift-and-scrape technique that entails the creation of a smaller flap and the subsequent removal of enough peripheral epithelium to allow for flap stretching. This avoids potential problems associated with epithelial overlap while at the same time improving the ease of flap creation.

## Introduction

Laser-assisted subepithelial keratectomy (LASEK) is an effective keratorefractive surface-ablation procedure for the correction of myopia, hyperopia, and astigmatism.[1,2,3,4,5,6] During the LASEK procedure, a dilute ethyl alcohol solution is applied to the corneal surface to loosen the epithelium, and microsurgical instruments are used to manually lift and reflect the hinged epithelial sheet away from Bowman's layer. After excimer laser ablation is performed, the epithelial flap is positioned back onto the treated stromal surface, where it remains during the first several postoperative days until complete epithelial regeneration has taken place.

The manipulation involved in reflecting and repositioning the epithelium often stretches the flap beyond its original dimensions, causing the flap edges to overlap the border of peripheral epithelium once the flap is repositioned. We believe that the presence of this overlapping epithelium may potentially interfere with the healing process and lead to increased patient discomfort and delayed visual recovery. This is partially based upon our experience with several cases of spontaneous epithelial sloughing after LASEK, all of which occurred shortly after bandage contact lens removal. In each of these cases, retained pieces of the epithelial flap were noted to be adherent to the newly regenerated epithelium, a finding which we believe may be associated with epithelial overlap.

We describe a technique that creates a smaller flap to allow for epithelial stretching while still maintaining the dimensions of the flap within the peripheral epithelial border. Two different sized epithelial trephines are used to create concentric grooves on the corneal surface. The epithelial flap, demarcated by the inner groove, is lifted in the standard fashion, after which the epithelium between the inner and outer grooves is removed. This "lift-and-scrape" technique provides a larger stromal surface to accommodate any stretching which may occur during flap manipulation.

## Surgical Technique

The eye is anesthetized, prepped, and draped in the standard fashion. An 8.0 mm LASEK epithelial trephine (Katena K2-7830) with a superior hinge is placed over the visual axis, decentered superiorly by one millimeter, and gently pressed onto the corneal surface with a slight twisting motion. A 9.0 mm trephine (Katena K2-7832) is then used to create a second groove that encompasses the first trephination groove but maintains the hinge in the same position as the 8.0 mm trephine. This creates a crescent-shaped pattern with a 90-degree gap between the points of the crescent (Figure 1).

A 9.5 mm holding well is then placed on the cornea to encircle the outer trephination groove and filled with an 18-20% ethyl alcohol solution. An alcohol application time of 30 seconds is used for the majority of these procedures. After the alcohol is absorbed with a surgical sponge, the cornea is rinsed with balanced salt solution (BSS®) and dried with another surgical sponge. A hinged epithelial flap is created with a combination micro-hoe/spatula (Katena K3-1848), using the inner 8.0 mm trephination groove as the flap outline (Figure 2). Once the flap is reflected, a micro-hoe is then used to scrape off the crescent-shaped area of epithelium remaining inside the 9.0 mm groove (Figure 3).

* Correspondence: Kraig S. Bower, MD FACS, Center for Refractive Surgery, Room 2F-205, Walter Reed Army Medical Center, 6900 Georgia Avenue NW, Washington, DC 20307-5001; Phone: 202-782-0202, Fax: 202-782-4653, Email: kraig.bower@ amedd.army.mil.

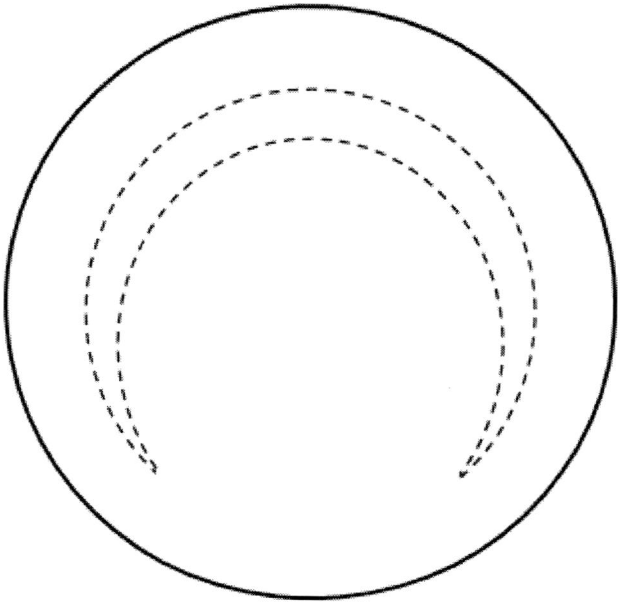

Figure 1. The 9.0 mm trephination groove encompasses the 8.0 mm trephination groove to form a crescent.

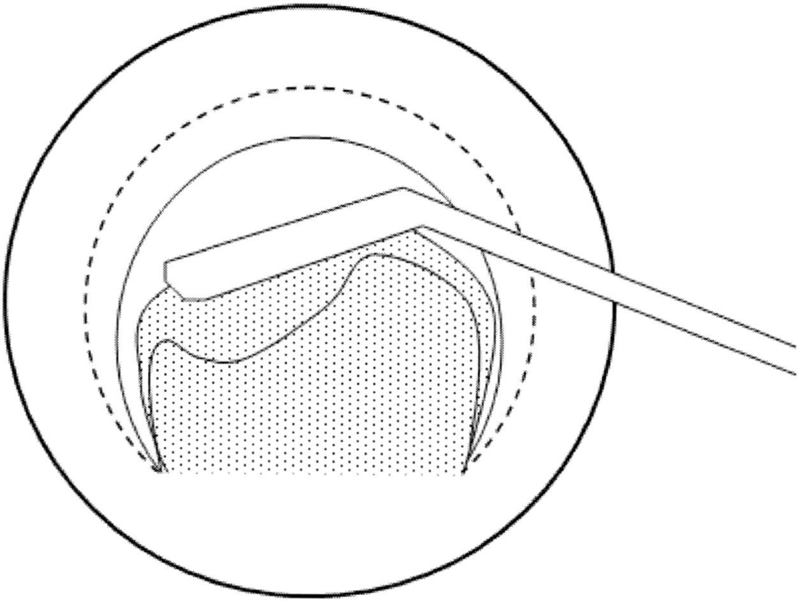

Figure 2. After alcohol application, the epithelial flap is created using the inner 8.0 mm trephination grcove as an outline.

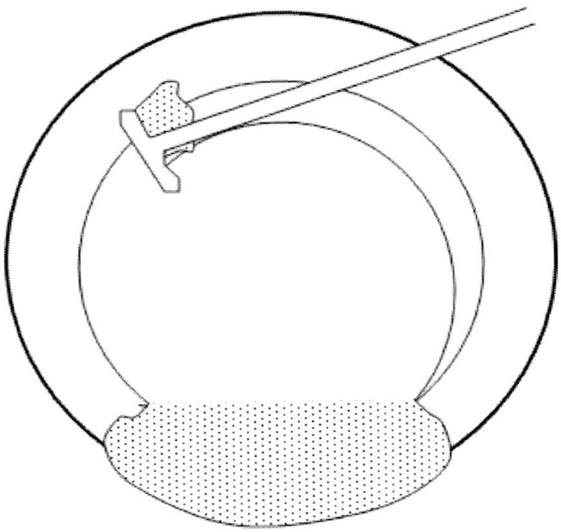

Figure 3. Once the flap is reflected, the epithelium remaining between the 8.0 and 9.0 mm trephination grooves is removed with a micro-hoe.

Stromal ablation is performed with the excimer laser, and the ablated surface is irrigated with chilled balanced salt solution (BSS®). The epithelial flap is then repositioned onto the stromal surface with a spatula or blunt cannula (Figure 4), taking care to align the flap edges within the borders of the peripheral epithelium.

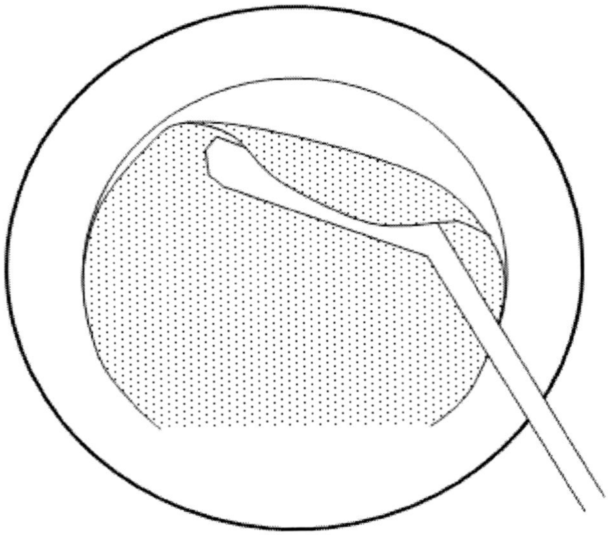

Figure 4. After excimer laser ablation is performed, the epithelial flap is repositioned over the treated stromal surface, taking care to align the flap edges within the border of peripheral epithelium.

Immediately following surgery, a bandage contact lens (Proclear Compatibles®, CooperVision, Norfolk, Virginia) is placed over the cornea, and topical antibiotic, steroid and non-steroidal eye drops are administered. The contact lens is left in place until the cornea re-epithelializes, which in most cases is complete by day four. Post-operative analgesia includes acetaminophen with codeine administered orally every 4 to 6 hours as needed, and topical diclofenac 0.1% ophthalmic solution (Voltaren®, Novartis Ophthalmics, Inc., Duluth, Georgia) up to four times per day for the first 3 days as needed. Moxifloxacin 0.5% topical ophthalmic solution (Vigamox®, Alcon Laboratories, Fort Worth, Texas) is administered four times per day for one week postoperatively then discontinued. The patient is instructed to use topical fluorometholone 0.1% suspension four times per day for the first two to four weeks, after which a one to three month taper is instituted based on the preoperative and postoperative refractive error, using the parameters described by Claringbold.[1]

# Results

Utilizing this technique, we have treated 298 eyes in 149 patients between -2.25 and -9.25 diopters. All treatments were performed at the Center for Refractive Surgery, Walter Reed Army Medical Center, Washington, DC, using the LADARVision™ excimer laser system (Alcon Surgical, Fort Worth, Texas) with Jupiter 2 software version 5.11. Comparison with the prior 187 LASEK cases performed by our service showed no statistically significant difference in pre- and postoperative vision and refractive error (Table 1). The incidence of intra-operative flap loss in the pre-modification group was 4 out of 187 (2.1%), compared to 1 out of 298 (0.3%) in the lift-and-scrape group (Table 1). This difference was statistically

**Table 1. Comparison of surgical results and complications**

| | Standard LASEK (n = 187) | Lift-and-scrape LASEK (n = 298) | *P* value |
|---|---|---|---|
| SE refraction, mean ± SD | | | |
| Preoperative | -5.16 ± 1.64 | -4.95 ± 1.29 | 0.11 |
| Postoperative (at final visit*) | -0.08 ± 0.30 | -0.04 ± 0.30 | 0.11 |
| Postoperative UCVA (at final visit*) | | | |
| 20/40 or better | 187 (100%) | 298 (100%) | N/A |
| 20/20 or better | 180 (96.3%) | 287 (96.3%) | 0.49 |
| Complications | | | |
| Lost flaps (intraoperative) | 4 (2.1%) | 1 (0.3%) | 0.03 |
| Epithelial sloughing (at 4 days) | 7 (3.7%) | 4 (1.4%) | 0.08 |
| Mean haze score** (at final visit*) | 0.23 | 0.22 | 0.73 |
| Loss of >1 line BCVA (at final visit*) | 0 | 0 | N/A |

* 3 - 6 months postop

** scale = 0 - 4

significant ($P$ = 0.02). There was small difference (3.7% vs. 1.4%) in the pre- and post-modification rates of spontaneous epithelial sloughing after BCL removal (Table 1), which approached but did not reach statistical significance ($P$ = 0.08). There were no cases of infectious keratitis or persistent epithelial defects beyond the first postoperative week. The mean haze score from both groups was virtually identical (Table 1), and no eyes from either group lost more than one line of final BCVA.

## Discussion

This simple modification of the LASEK technique is easy to adapt, requires no additional instrumentation, and adds a negligible amount of time to the total length of the procedure. We have found that this technique significantly reduces and in most cases eliminates intraoperative epithelial flap overlap. A potential concern is that a small gap is sometimes left between the flap edge and peripheral epithelium, but we have not found this to adversely affect the patient's comfort level or visual recovery in any way.

Before developing the lift-and-scrape technique, we observed occasional cases of spontaneous epithelial sloughing occurring on the fourth postoperative day. In each case, the patient presented minutes to hours after bandage contact lens removal with a spontaneous epithelial defect, despite visual confirmation of complete epithelial regeneration at the slit lamp. In all of these cases, it was also noted that pieces of redundant epithelium, presumably remnants of the LASEK flap, were adherent to the corneal surface immediately after contact lens removal. We believe that peripheral flap overlap may be responsible for these epithelial remnants, which could conceivably serve as a grasping point to "pull out the rug" from under the newly regenerated epithelium. Further investigation through prospective clinical trials will be necessary to determine whether the lift-and-scrape technique is associated with a statistically significant reduction in the incidence of this complication. It should be noted that all cases of epithelial sloughing were successfully treated with bandage contact lenses and topical antibiotics, and that all achieved a final UCVA of 20/20 or better.

Another potential benefit of this technique is that it appears to increase the ease of flap creation, partially due to the simple fact that a smaller flap is easier to lift. We have also observed that epithelial adhesion to Bowman's layer tends to be stronger towards the periphery of the cornea. Hence, initiating the flap edge more centrally decreases the manipulation required to lift the flap, and may also shorten the alcohol application time needed to loosen the epithelium. This can result in increased epithelial cell viability;[7,8] healthier and more reproducible flaps; and a smoother, less tedious, and potentially shorter surgical procedure.

Using the Alcon LADARVision 4000 excimer laser, we have found the above instrumentation to be ideal for spherocylindrical treatments, which incorporate a blend zone to produce an 8 to 9 mm ablation pattern. However, a 9.0 mm stromal surface is far larger than required to accommodate spherical treatments with a 6 to 7 mm ablation pattern. To our knowledge, there are no LASEK trephines smaller than 8.0 mm available that could be used to perform this technique for smaller ablation patterns. In these instances, we have adapted the lift-and-scrape technique by using a micro-hoe to free-hand a 7.0 mm flap inside an 8.0

mm trephination groove, thus limiting the size of the treatment area to the standard eight millimeters. In our experience, a 25-second alcohol application time provides sufficient epithelial loosening in the vast majority of these cases.

In 298 consecutive cases, we have not encountered any significant drawbacks in utilizing the lift-and-scrape technique. No additional equipment is required to adopt this modification, and no surgical risk is incurred beyond that seen in standard LASEK. While the potential benefits of eliminating flap overlap are largely theoretical at this point, we believe that the improved ease and reproducibility of flap creation are well worth the minimal time and effort it takes to adopt this technique.

# References

[1] Claringbold, T.V. Laser-assisted subepithelial keratectomy for the correction of myopia. *J Cataract Refract Surg*. 2002; 28:18-22.

[2] Shahinian, L., Jr. Laser-assisted subepithelial keratectomy for low to high myopia and astigmatism. *J Cataract Refract Surg.* 2002; 28:1334-1342.

[3] Anderson, N.J., Beran, R. and Schneider, T.L. Epi-LASEK for the correction of myopia and myopic astigmatism. *J Cataract Refract Surg.* 2002; 28:1343-1347.

[4] Autrata, R. and Rehurek, J. Laser-assisted subepithelial keratectomy and photorefractive keratectomy for the correction of hyperopia: Results of a 2-year follow-up. *J Cataract Refract Surg.* 2003; 29:2105-2113.

[5] Taneri, S., Feit, R. and Azar, D.T. Safety, efficacy, and stability indices of LASEK correction in moderate myopia and astigmatism. *J Cataract Refract Surg*. 2004; 30:2130-2137.

[6] Taneri, S., Zieske, J.D. and Azar, D.T. Evolution, techniques, clinical outcomes, and pathophysiology of LASEK: review of the literature. *Survey Ophthalmol.* 2004; 49:576-602.

[7] Chen, C.C., Chang, J.H., Lee, J.B., et al. Human corneal epithelial cell viability and morphology after dilute alcohol exposure. *Invest Ophthalmol Vis Sci.* 2002; 43:2593-2602.

[8] Gabler, B., Winkler von Mohrenfels, C., Dreiss, A.K., et al. Vitality of epithelial cells after alcohol exposure during LASEK flap preparation. *J Cataract Refract Surg*. 2002; 28:1841-1846.

Disclaimer: The opinions expressed in this manuscript are those solely of the authors and do not represent the views or official policies of the United States Army or Department of Defense.

In: Laser Keratectomy: Approaches, Complications...
Author: Luis W. Schröder and Felix J. Walter
ISBN 978-1-60456-863-9


*Chapter V*

# Surface Ablation Techniques: Photorefractive Keratectomy (PRK), Mitomycin-C (MMC) PRK, Laser Epithelial Keratomileusis (LASEK) and Epithelial Laser in Situ Keratomileusis (Epi-LASIK)

***Jayson D. Edwards and Kraig S. Bower***
Center for Refractive Surgery, Walter Reed Army Medical Center
Washington, DC, USA

## Abstract

The risk of postoperative flap dislocation, iatrogenic ectasia, epithelial ingrowth and other complications of laser in situ keratomileusis (LASIK) have led to renewed interest in surface ablation techniques. Photorefractive keratectomy (PRK) performed with and without the use of mitomycin-C (MMC), laser epithelial keratomileusis (LASEK) and epithelial laser in situ keratomileusis (Epi-LASIK) are all used extensively in the U.S. military. Research into the long term outcomes of surface ablation techniques is currently underway at Walter Reed Army Medical Center. In this paper we review the scientific rationale, indications, techniques, and outcomes for advanced surface ablations at Walter Reed Army Medical Center.

## Introduction

### History of Refractive Surgery

Though modern refractive surgery techniques have been developed over the past 30 years, attempts to correct nearsightedness without the use of glasses have been ongoing for centuries. Ancient Chinese reportedly placed sandbags over their eyes while sleeping to flatten their corneas as an attempt to improve their vision [1].

The first modern push towards non-spectacle vision correction began when Frans Cornelius Donders, a Dutch physician, systematically described the anomalies of accommodation and their optical and clinical aspects in 1864 [2]. His report started the first movement to surgically correct refractive error. Several techniques were attempted, from simply removing healthy lenses to removing the vitreous, often with disastrous results, all in an attempt to change the refractive power or length of the axis of the eye. During this time, Dr. J. Ball promoted a device to "restore eyesight and render spectacles useless" [3]. This device consisted of a small, spring-loaded mallet mounted on an eye cup. It reportedly restored sight by pounding the cornea flat by striking it through a closed eyelid. Charles Tyrrell aggressively marketed his Ideal Sight Restorer, which was composed of a U-shaped device with eye cups and a rubber bulb at the base that purportedly improved vision by massaging the eyes [4].

A more scientific method towards developing a viable method of refractive surgery began in 1898 with Dutch physican Leendert Jan Lans [5]. Working on his doctorate, Lans published the results of experiments on rabbits to treat astigmatism using keratectomy, keratotomy and themokeratoplasty [6]. He found that the cornea could flatten in the perpendicular meridian when a transverse incision was made. He concluded that the incision would have to be deep to have any effect, and this effect would often be lost as the incision healed.

In 1936 Tsutomu Sato observed corneal flattening in a keratoconus patient due to spontaneous breaks in Descemet's membrane [7]. Three years later he developed a technique to cure keratoconus, astigmatism and myopia though anterior and posterior incisions of the cornea [8]. Though the incisions worked to change the corneal curvature and improve visual acuity, the posterior incisions disrupted the endothelium. Unfortunately, the corneal endothelium's role in maintaining clarity had not been elucidated at the time, and most of his patients later developed bullos keratopathy [9].

Sato's pioneering work was further developed by Svyatoslov Fyodorov of the Soviet Union. Fyodorov first learned of Sato's research and surgical techniques while attending the Japanese Ophthalmologic Conference in Niigata, Japan in 1960. It wasn't until 1972, when Fyodorov treated a 16 year old patient with corneal lacerations from shattered glasses, that he made a breakthrough in keratotomy. He found that precise, radial cuts at the anterior cornea, determined by a mathematical formula he devised to adjust to various corneal curvatures, provided him the ability to control the amount of visual correction [10].

Radial keratotomy was the first refractive procedure to gain widespread acceptance among the medical field. In the meantime, the excimer laser was being developed as a precursor to today's modern refractive surgical techniques.

## The Excimer Laser

The first use of a laser in refractive surgery was done by Beckman and associates in 1980 using a carbon dioxide laser. However, corneal changes were transient and other lasers and techniques were examined. The eximer laser, originally developed in 1975 [11-12], was found to be superior due to its ability to provide high energy to tissue without excessive thermal damage. John Taboada was the first to use the eximer laser on corneal tissue in 1981 [13], with Trokel [14] and associates reporting in 1983 that the laser was able to ablate anterior corneal tissue predictably without damage to surrounding structures. The 193-nm argon-fluorine eximer laser, as shown by Kruger et al. [15-16], produced a smoother, more precise ablation compared to longer wavelength lasers under development.

Excimer, derived from "excited" and "dimer", describes the energy source of the laser, in which electrical energy excites argon-flourine atoms, which emit photons of light. The excimer laser operates under the concept of photoablation, in that the UV energy of the laser exceeds that of molecular covelent bonds, initiating a photochemical process [17]. Under this energy insult, the breaking chemical bonds cause an increase in pressure and eject the molecular fragments [18-19]. Higher wavelengths were found to work through a photothermal process, causing increased damage to surrounding tissue. The short 193-nm wavelength, with low repetition pulses, is able to remove tissue with very little local thermal damage [20]. The amount of tissue removed is proportional to the amount of energy that is delivered to the cornea.

Two types of delivery systems are available for the excimer laser: broad-beam and small spot scanning lasers. The broad beam approach – also known as variable-beam fixed spot (VFS) – employs a diaphragm delivery system that acts similarly to a camera to change the aperture. This can be done by use of an iris diaphragm or variable aperture system. This method of delivery has the advantage of fast treatment times, lessening fixation loss, corneal dehydration and patient discomfort. However, the diaphragm approach also results in "step-like" ablation patterns, which is believed to result in a more aggressive healing response [21].

Small spot scanning delivery can be subdivided into flying spot and rectangular beam scanning. The beams created are small (0.2 to 1 mm), allowing versatility in patterns to alter the topography of the cornea over large treatment zones. The small beam is more homogenous and allows for overlapping and multidirectional scanning, which results in a smoother ablation profile [22-23]. The flying spot technique can be customized to achieve virtually any ablation pattern by computer controlled "pixel-by-pixel" corneal ablations [21]. This variability also allows treatment of hyperopia, asymmetrical astigmatism, and phototheraputic keratectomy (PTK). Another advantage of scanning delivery systems is that an area of the cornea is not exposed to the laser continuously, so the temperature of the corneal tissue is lower than in broad-beam lasers. The small spot delivered allows for a smaller energy source and fewer optics, though the small amount of cornea ablated also results in longer treatment times. Corneal dehydration can occur, which increases the possibility of an uneven ablation [24]. Also, patient drift tends to increase due to longer treatment times. Active eye tracking systems are used to compensate for this drift.

## Photorefractive Keratectomy

The first refractive surgery technique to make use of the excimer laser system was photorefractive keratectomy (PRK) for treatment of myopia. Seiler of Germany was the first ophthalmologist to use the excimer laser for PRK ablations on humans [25]. The eyes used were blind or were to be enucleated. He followed this up later in 1987 with the first PRK ablation on a well-functioning eye [26]. L'Esperance was the first to perform PRK in the United States [27], and today the procedure is still considered an excellent technique with few serious complications. Though currently not as popular as laser in situ keratomileusis (LASIK), PRK is advantageous in its reliable safety and predictability in low to moderate myopes. Higher myopic correction is limited by increased corneal haze, pain and myopic regression [28-31].

## Indications for PRK

The decision to undergo refractive surgery rests with the patient, as does the choice of which procedure to receive. LASIK is the most common refractive surgery today, though the number of PRK procedures is increasing. Many patients are now opting for surface ablation procedures over LASIK due to excellent visual outcomes and a better safety profile. LASIK complications that are of concern include postsurgical traumatic flap dislocations, free caps, incomplete or irregular flaps, flap wrinkles or striae, buttonholes, flap melts, diffuse lamellar keratitis, corneal ectasia, epithelial defects, epithelial ingrowth and microbial keratitis [32-41]. PRK, however, is not without its complications, many of which LASIK is able to overcome. PRK complications include subepithelial haze, a lengthened recovery time and postoperative discomfort.

PRK is preferred in patients that have a history of recurrent erosions or anterior basement membrane dystrophies, as LASIK can exacerbate these conditions [42]. Lee and associates found that patients receiving PRK had a decreased incidence of postsurgical dry eye than in patients that underwent LASIK [43]. Patients that have low myopia, and as such low risk of haze formation may also do better with PRK. Additionally, PRK can be used in patients that have had previous surgery, such as radial keratectomy or LASIK [44].

In LASIK a hinged flap 80 to 200 μm is created using a microkeratome. In order to create this flap a suction ring is used on the eye, which temporarily results in an intraocular pressure (IOP) that can be greater than 65 mm Hg. PRK is recommended for glaucoma patients as the increased pressure of the suction ring in LASIK is contraindicated. In addition, patients that have deep orbits, poor exposure or anteriorly placed scleral buckles are more likely to have complications induced during flap creation. Patients with thin corneas in which the residual bed thickness under a LASIK flap is less than 250-300 μm, flat corneas (40 diopters or less) or very steep corneas (48 to 50 diopters) are best managed with PRK. In addition, patients at risk of corneal ectasia from forme fruste keratoconus or asymmetric astigmatism are also better PRK candidates [45].

Lifestyle must also be considered, as patients that are active in contact sports or in the military are at risk for postoperative flap dislocation after LASIK. Finally, a surgeon's experience should also be taken into account, as those that perform refractive surgery infrequently may be better with the less complicated PRK procedure [46].

## Surgical Technique

The goal of PRK is to change of the change the shape of the cornea, thus eliciting a change in its refractive power. This is accomplished in a two-step process – removal of the epithelium and laser treatment of the stroma.

Epithelial removal can be accomplished several different ways – mechanical, chemical or laser removal. Mechanical removal entails using a surgical blade or a rotating brush. Using a blade or spatula has been employed since the early days of surface ablation. Scraping the epithelium with a blade is carefully done, starting with the periphery to protect the central corneal and prevent dehydration. However, it may leave an irregular border or nicks in Bowman's layer. Alternatively, an Amoils or Pallikaris brush may be used to brush away the epithelium. Epithelial debris is wiped from the exposed stroma with a moistened sponge or spatula.

The basis of chemical removal of the epithelium is to disrupt the demosomes and hemidesmosomes that anchor the epithelial cells together. Several chemicals have been used to achieve this, including proparacaine, tetracaine, iodine, cocaine, lidocaine and n-heptanol. Topical anesthetics were effective, but took several minutes to work. Today 18-20% ethanol, which takes only 15 to 20 seconds, is the most commonly used chemical for epithelial debridement. In this technique the ethanol is either placed in a well or soaked in a sponge which is positioned on the cornea. This rapidly loosens the epithelium, which can then be scraped away. However, alcohol can be toxic to the epithelium and stroma as well as dehydrate the cornea.

Removal of the epithelium can also be done by the excimer laser in a process called transepithelial ablation. The central epithelium is approximately 50 μm thick and can be ablated under cobalt blue fluorescence. When the epithelium is removed and Bowman's layer exposed the fluorescence dissipates. However, the endpoint of epithelial removal is difficult to determine visually and there is variability of thickness of the epithelium over the cornea, which may lead to over or under ablation. Many practitioners have adopted laser scrape it its stead, in which the epithelium is deliberately ablated to a thickness of 40 μm, and the remaining basal layer is removed by mechanical debridement.

Since the first PRK procedure, laser technology and software have evolved and improved. The size of the ablation zone has also increased. To minimize the depth of ablation, the ablation zone initially was 3.5 to 4 mm. However, that caused edge glare and light sensitivity, especially at night. The ablation zone now is designed to be larger than the patient's fully dilated pupil, usually 5 to 8 mm, with smoothing of the edge at the transition zone. Ablation is then done in this area in a multizone/multipass technique in order to decrease corneal heating and provide a smoother ablation contour. Central corneal ablations are done in myopic patients, and peripheral ablations in hyperopic patients. A cross-cylinder ablation has been successful in patients with astigmatism.

Postoperatively, patients received a bandage contact lens that protects the de-epithelialized cornea. Lenses are generally worn for 4 to 5 days to reduce pain and aid the healing process. High oxygen permeable contact lenses are gaining greater use as they have been shown to result in faster corneal re-epithelialization and decreased pain (unpublished results). The postoperative epithelial defect increases susceptibility to bacterial keratitis, so topical antibiotics are provided. These are generally fluoroquinolones, which have broad spectrum coverage and excellent ocular tolerance [47]. Topical steroids are also provided to patients as the damaged stromal cells release cytokines, decreasing the incidence of sterile infiltrates and subepithelial haze.

## Complications of Wound Healing and Current Treatments

Though intraoperative and postoperative complications associated with PRK are uncommon, the increased incidence in corneal haze is of particular concern, especially in patients with higher degrees of myopia (greater than -6.00 diopters). Early haze formation is generally associated with wound healing, while late onset haze has been found to have a strong correlation to increased sensitivity to ultraviolet light following PRK. In addition, post-surgical regression is thought to be influenced by wound healing.

Epithelial wound healing occurs immediately after refractive surgery, controlled by cytokine mediators produced from stromal keratocytes and fibroblasts as well as lacrimal growth factors, such as tear fluid transforming growth factor-β1 (TGF- β1) 1[48-149]. Normally protected by the overlying epithelium, the corneal stroma responds to these lacrimal-gland derived growth factors, causing the activation and proliferation of keratocytes and resultant differentiation of fibroblasts and myofibroblasts. Each of these cell types participates in corneal haze. Preoperative keratocytes have a very low reflectivity of light. Following laser ablation, the keratocytes in the ablation zone become activated and highly reflective [50]. Fibroblasts and myofibroblasts also contribute to corneal haze due to their opacity [51]. In addition, the collagen produced by myofibroblasts is highly disorganized, lacking the ordered structure needed for transparency [52-53]. Patients with higher myopic correction require deeper ablation, resulting in a larger number of activated keratocytes, and a strong correlation between the degree of myopia and the degree of haze formation [54-55].

Epithelial hyperplasia has been shown to occur in both PRK [56] and LASIK [57], resulting in myopic regression. It is believed that this hyperplasia is associated with high levels of cytokines produced from corneal keratocytes, fibroblasts and myofibroblasts. Hepatocyte growth factor (HGF) and keratinocyte growth factor (KGF) are thought to be these modulators of epithelial proliferation [58]. This epithelial hyperplasia can be permanent.

Topical corticosteroids are often used postoperatively to treat both haze and regression. It is not clear, however, if steroids actually decrease the incidence of haze, and prolonged used can lead to adverse effects such as increases in intraocular pressure, band keratopathy and cataracts. Some studies have shown no benefit from steroids, others have shown a transient effect on haze that lasts only until steroids are discontinued [59-61].

The use of Mitomycin-C (0.02%) has been advanced as a solution in prevention and treatment of corneal haze by inhibiting the activation of keratocytes, resulting in decreased formation of haze. Phototheraputic keratectomy (PTK) and corneal scraping are used as treatments for haze formation, though the haze often recurs. Using mitomycin-C as an adjunct to these treatments has been effective in preventing haze from returning. In a study by Vigo et al. 100% of eyes that had developed moderate to severe haze following PRK showed improvement, up to 6 lines, in best corrected visual acuity following scraping and treatment with 0.02% mitomycin-C for 2 minutes [62]. Raviv et al. reported improvement in best corrected and uncorrected visual acuity in all 30 eyes treated with mitomycin-C after post-PRK haze formation [63]. In addition to treatment, mitomycin-C has also been shown to prevent haze formation. In a study of 60 eyes treated with PRK, 30 eyes were immediately treated with mitomycin-C. None of the 30 eyes treated with mitomycin-C developed more than trace haze, while 19 of the control eyes developed mild to severe haze [64].

Additional treatments of corneal haze include oral ascorbic acid prophylaxis and topical thiotepa. Ascorbic acid has been found to diminish an excessive wound response by decreasing keratocyte activation and protecting against UV damage [65-166]. Thiotepa, an antineoplastic agent, has been shown to successfully reduce haze in patients who didn't respond to conventional treatment [67].

## Laser Subepithelial Keratomileusis

Though LASIK is by far the most popular photorefractive technique used today, surface ablation techniques have again gained interest as surgeons endeavor to overcome the complications of creating a corneal flap. Laser subepithelial keratomileusis (LASEK), first described by Massimo Camellin [68] in 1999, is a modification of PRK in which dilute ethanol is used to loosen the epithelial adhesions from the underlying Bowman's layer. In contrast to PRK, the epithelium is repositioned following laser ablation.

## Indications

LASEK, in theory, incorporates the most beneficial aspects of both PRK and LASIK. As it is a surface ablation procedure, its safety and predictability profile are similar to PRK. There is no intrastromal incision so the technique does not suffer from flap complications seen in LASIK. The repositioned epithelial flap decreases both the amount of postoperative pain and the potential for the development of corneal haze by cytokine mediators, two significant drawbacks to PRK [69].

The most ideal candidates are those with mild to moderate myopia up to -7.00 diopters, thin corneas, anterior basement membrane disease, individuals involved in contact sports or the military, and other indications similar to PRK. However, LASEK incorporates the advantages of LASIK, including reduced postoperative pain and corneal opacities, rapid visual recovery and faster stabilization of refractive regression. The differences between LASEK, PRK and LASIK are only observed in the first few weeks, with long term visual outcome similar in all three techniques.

## Surgical Technique

There are several different techniques that can be used in LASEK, all derived from the used of chemical epithelial removal seen in PRK. The first technique used was the Camellin technique [68], which begins with a pre-cut epithelial trephination that allows greater access of the ethanol to the basement membrane. The trephine has a 90 degree blunt area at the 12 o'clock position for the hinge. A holding well is placed on the cornea and filled with 18 to 20% ethanol solution for 25 to 30 seconds. The cornea is rinsed and a spatula used to reflect the epithelial flap.

The Azar technique begins with labeling the cornea with overlapping 3 mm circles for positioning [70]. A semi-sharp well is place on the cornea and filled with ethanol, after which a modified Vannas scissors is used peripherally to cut the flap. The epithelial flap can then be peel back using a Merocel sponge.

Vinciguerra developed his technique in order to preserve epithelial attachment to the limbal stem cells [71]. Called the butterfly technique, a paracentral cut is made instead of a peripheral cut. This cut allows the formation of two flaps, which can then be reflected back to expose the stroma.

McDonald's technique [72] the does not require the use of ethanol and is loosely based off the butterfly technique. After trephination, a cataract blade is used to score the epithelium peripherally down to Bowman's layer. Viscous gel can then be injected under the epithelium, elavating the flap. A paracentral cut is then made with Vannas scissors and the two flaps resected back.

The purpose of any of these techniques is to expose the corneal stroma for laser ablation. The epithelial flap, retained with a hinge, can then be placed back into position and a bandage contact lens fit upon completion.

## Ethanol Toxicity

The major detrimental factor of LASEK procedures stems from the toxicity of ethanol to the corneal epithelium. Cell viability is determined by ethanol concentration and exposure time. Previous studies have determined that a concentration of 20% ethanol placed on the cornea for 20 seconds causes death in about 20% of cells. After 30 seconds of exposure 30% of the cells were dead and after 40 seconds 90% were dead [73]. Though the current protocol allows for 80% of the cells to be retained, there is still concern for the overall viability of the epithelial flap. Whether the flap readheres to the stroma, or simply acts as biological bandage until new epithelium grows in its stead is still a subject of debate.

## Epithelial Laser in Situ Keratomileusis (Epi-LASIK)

Epi-LASIK, a variation of LASEK, has recently emerged in an effort to combat the risk of ethanol toxicity to the corneal epithelium and stroma. First described by Ioannis Pallikaris

[74], this technique incorporates the use of a microkeratome-like device that mechanically separates the epithelial cells from Bowman's layer.

### Indications

Patient selection for those receiving Epi-LASIK is similar to other surface ablation profiles. Proponents of this technique state that healing times and haze formations are decreased compared to PRK. Candidates are those with low to moderate myopia, thinner corneal thickness, steep or flat corneas or other contraindications of LASIK. Ethanol is not used for the creation of the epithelial flap and has no inherent risk or complication of ethanol toxicity seen in LASEK. Additionally, some patients may express anxiety towards a corneal stromal cut of LASIK, and the bladeless technique of Epi-LASIK can be an alternative.

### Surgical Technique

Mechanical exposure of the stroma is the defining feature of Epi-LASIK. A modified microkeratome is used to create the epithelial flap. This epimicrokeratome uses a suction ring and a blunt oscillating seperator to detach the epithelium, leaving a 2 to 3 mm nasal hinge. The epithelial flap can then be reflected back and laser ablation done on the stroma. A bandage contact lens is placed postoperatively. Designed to eliminate the complications of ethanol exposure, the Epi-LASIK microkeratome is supposed to preserve the basement membrane by placing the cleavage plane beneath it. However, due to variability of eyes, the cleavage plane has been inconsistent with reports of microfocal damage to the lamina densa [75].

## Surface Ablations at Walter Reed Army Medical Center

ThoughWhile LASIK is the most popular method in most corneal refractive surgery practices, most military personnel do not qualify for LASIK due to the risk of traumatic postoperative flap dislocation, and in general undergo surface ablation procedures. PRK is the most common surface ablation techniques used in the military [76]. However, concerns over post-PRK haze have lead refractive surgeons to find alternative surface ablation techniques. Several small case series, clinical trials and anecdotal experiences suggest that there is a lower incidence of haze associated with mitomycin C PRK (MMC PRK) and LASEK than there is with PRK. An ongoing prospective clinical study at the Walter Reed Army Medical Center's Center for Refractive Surgery is underway to determine differences in visual outcomes among the three procedures and to help standardize care.

# Patients and Methods

A total of 167 patients (334 eyes) underwent surface ablation treatment. Patients were randomized to treatment of their dominant eye with either MMC PRK (0.1 mg/ml x 1 minute) or LASEK. The fellow eye received conventional PRK. Inclusion criteria included age 21 or above, manifest refractive spherical equivalent between -4.00 diopters and -10.00 diopters, refractive stability and best spectacle corrected visual acuity (BACVA) of 20/20 or better in both eyes. Exclusion criteria included female subjects who are pregnant who intend to become pregnant, residual, recurrent or active ocular disease, any medical condition that may impair healing, such as collagen vascular disease, autoimmune disease, ocular herpes infections or immunodeficiency disease, and current use of topical or systemic medications that impair healing, including corticosteroids, antimetabolites, etc.

All individuals received surface ablation using LADARVision™ excimer laser system (Alcon Surgical, Ft. Worth, Texas). Patients received topical tetracoine 0.5% prior to treatment. Eyes undergoing PRK (n = 167) or MMC PRK (n = 85) had the corneal epithelium removed with the used of an Amoils rotary brush. Eyes that underwent LASEK had a 9.0 mm flap created by use of a trephine, in which the hinge was positioned superiorly. The epithelial flap was loosened using 20% ethanol for 25 to 35 seconds and reflected superiorly using a spatula. After surface ablation, eyes receiving MMC PRK had a cornea light shield soaked with 0.02% mitomycin-C placed on the ablation zone and left in place for 60 seconds, after which the cornea was irrigated with one 30 ml bottle of chilled BSS. All eyes received postoperative moxifloxacin 0.5% and ketoralc 0.5% with placement of a bandage soft contact lens.

Patients returned for postoperative care at 1 day, 4 days and 1 week, with follow up examinations at 1, 3, 6 and 12 months. Visual outcomes measurements were taken at follow up visits, including uncorrected visual acuity (UCVA), best spectacle corrected visual acuity (BSCVA), manifest refraction, and 5% and 25% low contrast visual acuity (LCVA). Endothelial cell counts were assessed at 6 ant 12 months. UCVA and BSCVA measurements were taken using a 4 meter LogMAR back-illuminated eye chart (Lighthouse Second edition, New York, NY). A standardized phoropter with a vertex distance of 12.5 mm was used to evaluate manifest refraction. LCVA was assessed with the Precision Vision Optical series of LogMAR charts with back illumination at 5% and 25% contrast. Haze rate was recorded on a scale of 0 to 4. Endothelial cell counts were assessed with the ConfoScan4 confocal microscope (Nidek Technologies, Albignasego, Italy).

Results were recorded using an Excel spreadsheet (Microsoft Corp, Redmont, Washington), and data were analyzed using SPSS for Windows version 15.0 (SPSS Inc., Chicago, Illinois) using Mann-Whitney tests. A P values of $<0.5$ was considered statistically significant.

# Results

A total of 167 eyes underwent PRK, 84 eyes underwent MMC PRK and 83 eyes underwent LASEK. The mean patient age was 35 (range 21 to 57), with 57 female and 110 male patients. The preoperative mean spherical equivalent was -5.61 ±1.44 D (range 2.75 to -9.25 D), mean cylinder was -0.78 ±0.69 D (range 0 to -3.25 D) and mean manifest spherical equivalent was -6.00 ±1.42 D (range -3.88 to -9.38 D).

## Safety

The number of eyes losing two or more lines of BSCVA was used as a measurement of safety. At one month 4.3% of PRK, 4.8% of MMC PRK and 2.4% of LASEK eyes lost two or more lines BSCVA. At 3 months 1 PRK eye and 1 MMC PRK eye continued to have 2 or more lines lost of BSCVA. One patient that received PRK in one eye and LASEK in the other lost 3 lines bilaterally at 6 months due to 2+ corneal haze. One additional PRK eye lost 3 lines BSCVA at the 12 month post-op visit due to 2+ late onset corneal haze. The patient's alternate eye underwent LASEK and gained one line of BSCVA. This patient had no previous complications prior to 12 months. Both patients with late onset haze were treated with corneal scraping and MMC, with resolution of the haze and improvement in visual acuity to 20/20 or better.

## Efficacy

Efficacy was measured by UCVA of 20/20 and 20/40 and better. Results are shown in Figure 1. At one month more LASEK eyes (64.6%) compared to MMC PRK eyes (43.3%) had a postoperative visual acuity of 20/20 ($p=0.006$). Differences between groups were insignificant after 1 month.

Comparing pre-operative BSCVA with post-operative UCVA also provides a valuable test to evaluate efficacy. At one month postoperatively, UCVA was within one line of the pre-op BSCVA in 66.2% of LASEK eyes compared to 51.8% of MMC PRK eyes ($p = 0.12$). There was no significant difference between groups after the first post-operative month (Figure 2).

## Predictability

Predictability was at 1, 3, 6 and 12 months. While there was a trend towards better predictability of MMC PRK compared to either PRK or LASEK at one and 6 months postoperatively, there was no difference between the groups at the 12 month postoperative visit (Table 1).

## Quality of Vision

There were no statistically different changes between the three groups when measuring postoperative 5% LCVA and 25% LCVA. There was a trend towards improved 5% contrast in LASEK compared to PRK (p = 0.096) and MMC PRK (p = 0.075) at 3 months.

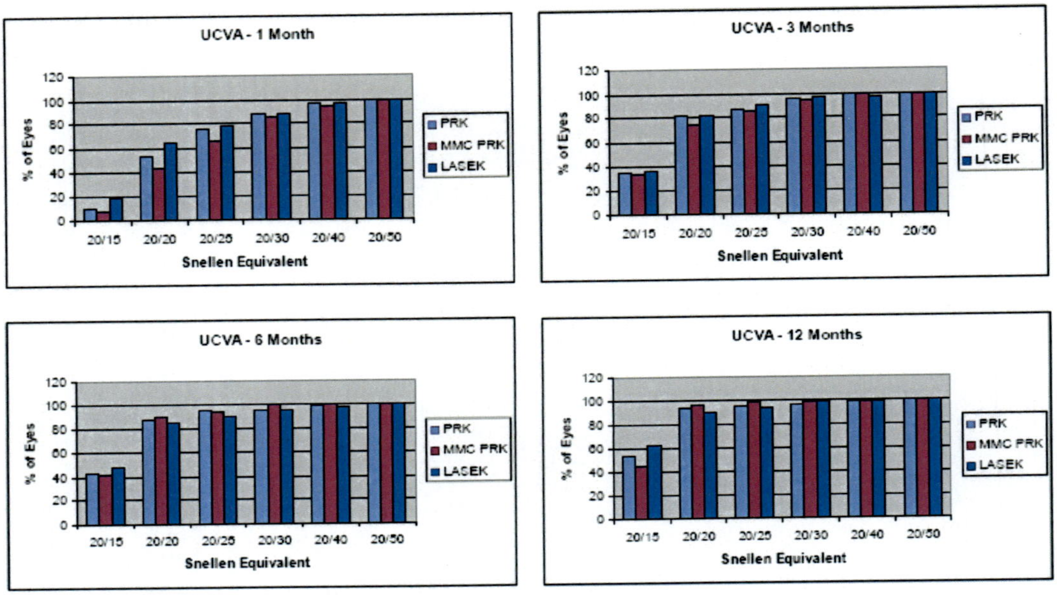


Figure 1. UCVA.

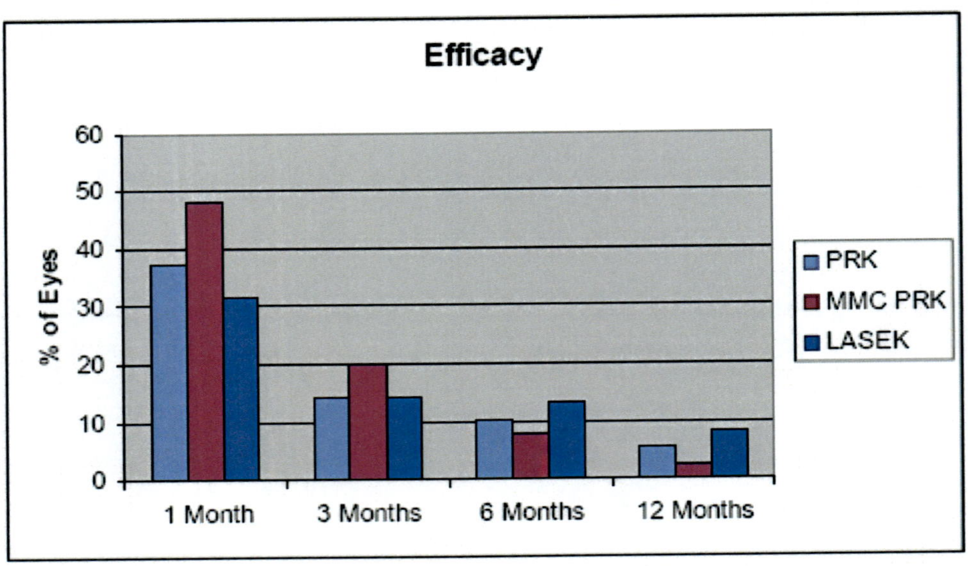


Figure 2. PreBSCVA vs PostUCVA eye with 2 or greater line loss.

## Corneal Haze

At the one month preoperative visit, more haze was present in LASEK eyes compared to both PRK (p = 0.021) and MMC PRK (p = 0.004). The only eye that had haze of grade 2 was in the LASEK group. No eye in any group was grades 3 or 4. All other eyes were grade 1.

**Table 1. Predictability. Goal to emmetropia, percentage of eyes**

| | PRK | | MMC PRK | | LASEK | |
|---|---|---|---|---|---|---|
| | ±0.5D | ±1.0D | ±0.5D | ±1.0D | ±0.5D | ±1.0D |
| 1 Month | 44.8 | 73.3 | 56.6 | 84.3 | 46.3 | 76.8 |
| 3 Months | 57.3 | 80.0 | 58.3 | 86.1 | 58.4 | 79.2 |
| 6 Months | 64.9 | 85.5 | 82.5 | 92.1 | 69.1 | 82.4 |
| 12 Months | 81.5 | 96.7 | 86.4 | 95.5 | 81.6 | 91.7 |

**Table 2. Percentage of eyes with haze. No eye developed grade 3 or 4 haze. Grade 2 haze was only found in one LASEK eye at 1 month and 1 PRK eye at 6 and 12 months. All other haze was grade 1**

| | 1 Month | 3 Months | 6 Months | 12 Months |
|---|---|---|---|---|
| PRK | 13.3 | 10.7 | 7.7 | 5.4 |
| MMC PRK | 8.4 | 4.1 | 1.6 | 2.3 |
| LASEK | 25.6 | 19.3 | 7.4 | 4.2 |

LASEK continued to have a statistically significant increase in haze at 3 months compared to MMC PRK (p = 0.005), though no eyes at 3 months were grade 2 or higher. There was no statistical significance between groups at 6 or 12 months. One PRK eye at both 6 and 12 months had haze of grade 2, all other eyes in all groups with haze were grade 1. Total percentages of eyes with haze, both grades 1 and 2, can be seen in Table 2.

## Endothelial Cell Counts

Endothelial cell counts were done preoperatively and at 6 months and 12 months as a determinant of corneal health following refractive surgery. For the PRK group there was found to be a median loss of 37 cells/mm2 (range -1092 to 633) at 6 months postoperatively and 94 cells/mm2 (range -682 to 890) at 12 months. This change was statistically significant at 12 months (p – 0.001). For the MMC PRK group there was a median loss of 55 cells/mm2 (range -574 to 672) at 6 months and 35 cells/mm2 (-605 to 882) at 12 months, neither of which was statistically significant (p = -0.344 and 0.429 respectively). Additionally, there was no significant change for the LASEK group with a median loss of 17 cells/mm2 (range -936 to 546) at 6 months and a median gain of 37 cells/mm2 (range -789 to 791) at 12 months (p = 0.911 and 0.259 respectively). There was a significant difference between the 3 groups at 12 months ($p = 0.021$). This difference was found to be primarily between the PRK and LASEK groups ($p = 0.004$).

## Epi-LASIK Results at Walter Reed Army Medical Center

Another novel surface ablation technique, Epi-LASIK, was developed in an attempt to improve upon the advantages of LASEK. By using mechanical separation of the epithelium from the underlying corneal stroma, it is anticipated that the resulting cell morphology and physiology will be more normal when compared to the chemical separation method used in LASEK. Several preliminary studies have shown it to be a safe and efficient treatment. An ongoing study at Walter Reed Center for Refractive Surgery is in progress to determine the short and long term affects of this new procedure.

## Patients and Methods

A total of 290 eyes of 145 active duty US Army soldiers, age 21 or over, received bilateral Epi-LASIK using the Amadeus™ II epikeratome and LADARVision™ 6000 excimer laser system. Patients were treated for myopia or myopic astigmatism with a manifest refractive spherical equivalent between -0.5 to -6.25 diopters.

The epikeratome parameters were set per the manufacturer's recommendation. Once the flap was created, it was moved superiorly with use of a microspatula, and photoablation was done on the underlying stroma. If there was a complication in the first eye (right eye) a new epithelial separator was used for the second eye. The epithelial flap was retained after laser ablation whenever possible. After laser ablation the epithelial flap was replaced and a bandage contact lens was applied.

Preoperative data included age, gender, MSE, refractive cylinder (CYL), keratometry (K) and central corneal thickness (CCT). Pain, corneal epithelium, UCVA and complications such as corneal infiltrates were assessed at 1 day, 4 days and 1 week postoperatively. UCVA, BSCVA, MSE and 5% and 25% LCVA were assessed at 1 and 3 month follow ups. The Epi-LASIK data were compared to an existing PRK data set that was collected under identical conditions.

Statistical analysis was performed using SPSS for Windows version 15.0. A Mann-Whitney test was used to compare UCVA and pain between Epi-LASIK and PRK. The Fisher's exact test was performed to assess the difference between the two groups when examining re-epithelialization and the presence of corneal infiltrates. A p-value of $<0.05$ was considered statistically significant. Odds ratios (OR) were used to determine likelihood of flap complications.

# Results

The mean age was 34 years old with 62.8% of patients male. The mean preoperative MSE was -2.93 +/- 1.19 D (range -1.00 to -6.25), mean cylinder was -0.56 +/- 0.51 D, K steep was 44.36 +/- 1.46 D, K flat was 43.55 +/- 1.44 D, and mean CCT was 540 +/- 34 μm.

**Table 3. Epi-LASIK flap complications, number of eyes and percentage**

| Complication | Number | Percent |
|---|---|---|
| No complication | 188 | 64.8 |
| Automatic flap amputation | 43 | 14.8 |
| Buttonhole flap | 17 | 5.9 |
| Hinge tear | 14 | 4.8 |
| Surgeon amputation (hinge in treatment zone) | 14 | 4.8 |
| Incomplete flap/ superficial resection | 8 | 2.8 |
| Stromal incursion | 6 | 2.1 |
| Total | 290 | 100.0 |

## Intraoperative Complications

An overview of the intraopertative complications can be seen in Table 3. Overall, there was a 35% chance of a flap complication, with a 23% chance of losing the flap. There was a relative increase in rate of complications for age ≤40 (OR = 1.33, P = 0.022), CCT < 500 μm (OR = 1.227, P = 0.590), right eye (OR = 1.53, P = -.085), K cylinder >1.0D (OR = 1.33, P = 0.288), and K flat <42.0D (OR = 1.21, P = 0.568). There was a decreased odds ratio for K steep >46.0D (OR = 0.568, P = 0.160).

**Table 3. Epi-LASIK intraoperative flap complications, number of eyes and percentage**


| Complication | Number | Percent |
|---|---|---|
| No complication | 188 | 64.8 |
| Automatic flap amputation | 43 | 14.8 |
| Buttonhole flap | 17 | 5.9 |
| Hinge tear | 14 | 4.8 |
| Surgeon amputation (hinge in treatment zone) | 14 | 4.8 |
| Incomplete flap/ superficial resection | 8 | 2.8 |
| Stromal incursion | 6 | 2.1 |
| Total | 290 | 100.0 |

### Early Healing Results

There was no statistical difference in pain scores between Epi-LASIK and PRK at any visit in the first week postoperatively. Re-epithelialization was significantly faster in PRK eyes, with 92% of PRK eyes compared to only 55.4% of Epi-LASIK eye fully healed by postoperative day 4 ($p = 0.000$), and 99% of PRK eyes compared to 88.5% of Epi-LASIK eyes fully healed by postoperative day 7 ($p = 0.000$). A total of 50 Epi-LASIK eyes and no PRK eyes required an additional visit at postoperative day 10 to assess completion of re-epithelialization.

### Long Term Healing Results

Epi-LASIK was associated with significantly worse UCVA at postoperative day 1 ($p = 0.002$) when compared to PRK. Otherwise, there was no other significant difference in UCVA, BSCVA or MSE up to 63 months postoperatively over time between groups. Efficacy was evaluated by comparing preoperative BSCVA to postoperative UCVA. Up to 3 months there was no statistical significance between the two groups. At 6 months efficacy in epi-LASIK patients was significantly better than in PRK patients, with 83.9% of epi-LASIK patients attaining a postoperative UCVA the same or better than preoperative BSCVA compared to 71.7% of PRK patients. There was no statistical difference in haze formation at 1, 3 and 6 month and 3 months. No eye developed grade 3 or 4 haze and only 2 Epi-LASIK eyes developed grade 2 haze at 1 month. All other haze at both 1, 3 and 6 and 3 months was grade 1 haze.

## Discussion

Though LASIK has only shown an advantage over surface ablation techniques during the first few weeks postoperatively [77-178], those early healing benefits have caused LASIK to flourish. LASEK and Epi-LASIK were developed to incorporate those advantages into the safety profile seen in PRK.

As the primary purpose of refractive surgery is to obtain the best visual acuity possible without the use of spectacles, assessing the visual outcomes is a determining factor in the success of a technique. Comparing preoperative BSCVA with postoperative UCVA is likely the main factor that a patient uses to determine the success of refractive surgery. In our study, at one month eyes receiving LASEK had a significantly better outcome than eyes receiving MMC PRK, with a trend towards improvement compared to PRK. Visual acuity after 1 month was equivalent between all three groups. This is in contrast to the study done by Ghadfan et al. [79], which showed a slightly better outcome with the PRK techniques compared to LASEK. MMC PRK, however, showed better predictability compared to both PRK and LASEK at one month.

There has been concern for acoustic or ultraviolet radiation damage on corneal endothelial cell density, as well as cytotoxic effects of mitomycin-C. Previous studies have shown no adverse effect on the clinical endothelium, both without [80] and in the presence of mitomycin-C [81]. Our results showed only a significant decrease in eyes receiving PRK at 12 months. There was no difference in endothelial cell density in eyes receiving MMC PRK or LASEK.

Our Epi-LASIK results are as yet incomplete to determine long-term visual outcomes, though uUp to three months there appeared to be no difference compared to PRK though at 6 months Epi-LASIK showed better efficacy than PRK. However, there has been concern for intraoperative complications of the Epi-LASIK flap. Over one-third of all patients had a flap complication, with 23% of all patients losing the flap. In addition, PRK eyes resulted in better postoperative healing, with faster re-epithelialization compared to Epi-LASIK eyes. Many patients that received Epi-LASIK also required an addition postoperative visit to assess healing and evaluate complications.

Haze has always been a concern in surface ablation procedures due to the loss of Bowman's layer and healing response. Previous studies have shown a decrease in haze in LASEK [82] and Epi-LASIK [83] compared to PRK, our studies showed worsening haze with LASEK. Haze rate was comparable among Epi-LASIK eyes and PRK eyes, providing support that the increased haze in LASEK eyes may have been related to the ethanol rather than the presence of a flap. This haze, however, was clinically insignificant, with clinically significant haze equivalent in both PRK and LASEK eyes.

## Conclusion

Though the advent of LASIK surgery was thought to be the death knoll for PRK, new surface ablations techniques such as LASEK and Epi-LASIK, advanced laser systems and an effort to avoid lamellar flap complications have given new breath to this venerable procedure. Until such time that outcomes of one technique proves superior to the others, no one technique will replace the others. In the U.S. military, surface ablation procedures are the principle refractive technique as the complications involved with a lamellar flap are greater in this active population. Continued research into new methods of reducing haze formation, decreasing postoperative pain, and improving on the safety, efficacy and predictability of surface ablations techniques will produce superior visual outcomes.

## References

[1] Leo D. Bores, Refractive Eye Surgery, 2nd Ed. Blackwell Science, Inc. Malden Massachusetts, 2001.

[2] Donders FC. On the Anomalies of Accommodation and Refraction of the Eye [translated by William D. Moore, M.D.]. London: New Sydenham Society, 1864.

[3] Podolsky, M. Lawrence, Cures Out of Chaos: How Unexpected Discoveries Led to Breakthroughs in Medicine and Health, Harwood Academic Publishers, 1998.

[4] AP Ferry, "Professor" Charles Tyrrell and his ideal sight restorer. *Ophthalmol.* 1986; 93:1246-57.

[5] Thornton SP. Background of incisional refractive surgery In: Wu HK, Thompson VM, et al, editors. Refractive Surgery New York: Thieme Medical Publishers, 1999:127–134.

[6] Lans LJ. Experimentelle Untersuchungen uber Entstehung von Astigmatismus durch night perforirende Corneawunden. *Arch. Ophthalmol.* 1898; 45:117-152.

[7] Sato T. Treatment of conical cornea (incision of Descemet's membrane). *Acta Soc. Ophthalmol. Jpn.* 1939; 43:544-555.

[8] Sato T, Akiyama K, Shibata H. A new surgical approach to myopia. *Am. J. Ophthalmol.* 1953; 36:823–829.

[9] Dawano H, Uesugi Y, Nakayasu K et al. Long-term follow up for bullous keratopathy after sato-type anterior-posterior corneal refractive surgery. *Am. J. Ophthalmol.* 2003; 136:1154-1155.

[10] Fyodorov SN, Durnev VV, Ivashina AI, Gudechkiv VB. Calculation method of effectiveness of anterior keratotomy in surgical correction of myopia. In Fyodorov SN (ed): Surgery for Anomalies in ocular Refraction. Moscow: The Moscow research institute for ocular Microsurgery. 1981, pp. 114-121.

[11] Krauss JM, Pauliafito CA steinert RF. Laser interactions with the cornea. *Surv. Ophthalmol.* 1986; 31:37-53.

[12] Seiler T. McDonnel PJ. Excimer laser photorefractive keratectomy. *Surv. Ophthalmol.* 1995; 40:89-118.

[13] Taboada J, Mikesell GW, Reed RD. Response of the corneal epithelium to KrF excimer laser pulses. *Healthe phys*. 1981; 40:677-683.

[14] Trokel SL, Srinivasan R, Braren B. Excimer laser surgery of the cornea. *Am. J. Ophthalmol.* 1983; 96:710-715.

[15] Krueger RR, Trokel SL, Schubert HD. Interaction of ultraviolet laser light with the cornea. *Invest Ophthalmol. Vis. Sci.* 1985; 26:1455-1464.

[16] Krueger RR, Trokel SL. Quantitation of corneal ablation by ultraviolet laser light. *Arch. ophthalmol.* 1985; 103:1741-1742.

[17] Keyes T, Clarke RH, Isner JM. Theory of photoablation and its implications for laser phototherapy. *J. Phys. Chem.* 1985; 89:4194-4196.

[18] Srinivasan R. Kinetics of ablative photodecompensation of organic polymers in the far-ultraviolet (193 nm). *J. Vac. Sci. Tech.* B 1983; 1:923-926.

[19] Puliafito CA, Stern D, Drueger RR, et al. High-speed photography of excimer laser ablation of the cornea. Arch Ophthalmol 1987; 105:1255-1259

[20] Puliafito CA, Wong K, Steinert RF. Quantitative and ultrastructural studies of excimer laser ablation of the cornea at 193 and 248 nanometers. *Lasers Surg. Med.* 1987; 7:155-159.

[21] Barnes S, Azar DT. Excimer laser surface ablation: Photorefractive keratectomy (PRK) and laser subepithelial keratomileusis (LASEK). In: Smolin G, Foster CF, Azar DT, et al, eds. Smolin and Thoft's The Cornea: Scientific Foundations and Clinical Practice, 4th Ed. Philadelphia: Lippincott Williams and Wilkins 2005;1182-1199.

[22] Campos M, Trokel SL, McDonnell PJ. Surface morphology following photorefractive keratectomy. *Ophthalmic Surg.* 1993; 24:822-825.

[23] Unkroth A, Kleinschmidt J, Ziegler W, et al. Ablation of the cornea by using a low-energy excimer laser. *Graefes Arch. Clin. Exp. Ophthalmol.* 1993; 231:303-307.

[24] Dougherty PJ, Wellish KL, Malony RK. Excimer laser ablation rate and corneal hydration. *Am. J. Ophthalmol.* 1994; 118:169-176.

[25] Seiler T, Wollensak J. In vivo experiments with the excimer laser – technical parameters and healing processes. *Ophthalomologica* 1986; 192:65-70.

[26] SeilerT, Wollensak J. Myopic photorefractive keratectomy with the excimer laser. One-year follow-up. *Ophthalmology* 1991; 98:1156-1163.

[27] L'Esperance FA, Taylor DM, Warner JW. Human excimer laser keratectomy: short-term histopathology. *Refract. Corneal Surg.* 1988; 96:654-664.

[28] O'Bart DPS, Corbett MC, Verma S, et al. Effects of ablation diameter, depth, and edge contour on the outcome of photorefractive keratectomy. *J. Refract. Surg* .1996; 12:50-60.

[29] Kim J,Woo S, Park C, Hahn T, Kim M. Myopic regression after photorefractive keratectomy. *Ophthalmi.c Surg. Lasers* 1996; 27:S435-439.

[30] Carson CA, Taylor HR. Excimer laser treatment for high and extreme myopia. *Arch. Ophthalmol.* 1995; 113:431–436.

[31] Braunstein RE, Jain S, McCally RI, et al. Objective measurement of corneal light scattering after excimer laser keratectomy. *Ophthalmol.* 1996; 103:439-443.

[32] Lin RT, Maloney RK. Flap complications associated with lamellar refractive surgery. *Am. J. Ophthalmol.* 1999; 127:129-136.

[33] Stulting DR, Carr JD, Thompson KP, et al. Complications of laser in situ keratomileusis for the correction of myopia. *Ophthalmol.* 1999; 106:13-20

[34] Al-Reefy M. Bacterial keratitis following laser in situ keratomileusis for hyperopia. *J. Refract. Surg.* 1999; 15:216-217.

[35] Wright JD Jr, Neubaur CC, Stevens G Jr. Epithelial ingrowth in a corneal graft treated by laser in situ keratuomileusis: light and electron microscopy. *J. Cataract. Refract. Surg.* 2000; 26:49-55.

[36] Castillo A, Diaz-Valle D, Gutierrez AR, et. al. Peripheral melt of flap after laser in situ keratomileusis. *J. Refract. Surg.* 1998; 14:61-63.

[37] Lombardo AJ, Katz HR. Late partial dislocation of a laser in situ keratomileusis flap. *J. Cataract. Refract. Surg.* 2001; 27:1108-1110.

[38] Leung AT, Rao SK, Lam DS. Traumatic partial unfolding of laser in situ keratomileusis flap with severe epithelial ingrowth. *J. Cataract. Refract. Surg.* 2000; 26:135-139.

[39] Melki SA, Talamo JH, Demetriades Am, et al. Late traumatic dislocation of laser in situ keratomileusis corneal flap. *Ophthalmol.* 2000; 107:2136-2139.

[40] Schwartz GS, Park DH, Schloff S, et al. Traumatic flap displacement and subsequent diffuse lamellar keratitis after laser in situ keratomileusis. *J. Cataract. Refract. Surg.* 2001; 27:781-783.

[41] Pallikaris IG, Kymionis GD, Astyrakakis NI. Corneal ectasia induced by laser in situ keratomileusis. *J. Cataract. Refract. Surg.* 2001; 27:1796-1802.

[42] Claringbold TV. Laser-assisted subepithelial keratectomy for the correction of myopia. *J. Cataract. Refract. Surg.* 2002; 28:18-22.

[43] LeeJB, Ryu CH, Kim J, et al. Comparison of tear secretion and tear film instability after photorefractive keratectomy and laser in situ keratomileusis. *J. Cataract. Refract. Surg.* 2000 26:1326-1331.

[44] Kohnen T. Retreating residual refractive errors after excimer surgery of the cornea: PRK versus LASIK. *J. Cataract. Refract. Surg.* 2000;25:625-626.

[45] Sun R, Gimbel HV, Kaye GB. Photorefractive keratectomy in keratoconus suspects. *J. Cataract. Refract. Surg.* 1999; 25:1461-1466.

[46] Yo C, Vroman D, Ma S, et al. Surgical outcomes of photorefractive keratectomy and laser in situ keratomileusis by inexperienced surgeons. *J. Cataract. Refract. Surg.* 2000; 26:510-515.

[47] Burka JM, Bower KS, VanRoekel RC, et al. The effect of moxifloxacin and gatifloxacin on long-term visual outcomes following photorefractive keratectomy. *J. Refract. Surg.* 2007; 23:414-417.

[48] Baldwin HC, Marshall J. Growth factors in corneal wound healing following refractive surgery: a review. *Acta Ophthalmol. Scand.* 2002; 80:238-247.

[49] Li DG, Tseng SC. Three patterns of cytokine expression potentially involved in epithelial-fibroblast interactions of human ocular surface. *J. Cell Physiol.* 2000; 27:565-570.

[50] Moller-Peterson T. Keratocyte reflectivity and corneal haze. *Exp. Eye Res.* 2004; 78:553-560.

[51] Jester JV, Petroll WM, Cavanagh HD. Corneal stromal wound healing in refractive surgery: the role of myofibroblasts. *Prog. Retin. Eye Res.* 1999; 18:311-356.

[52] Kaji Y, Obata H, usui T, et al. Three-dimensional organization of collagen fibrils during corneal stromal wound healing after excimer laser keratectomy. *J. Cataract Refract. Surg.* 1998; 24:1441-1446.

[53] Jester JV, Moller-Pederson T, Huang J, et al. The cellular basis of corneal transparency: evidence for corneal crystallins. *J. Cell Sci.* 1999; 112:613-622.

[54] Mohan rr, Hutcheon AEK, Choi R, et al. Apoptosis, necrosis, proliferation, and myofibroblast generation in the stroma following LASIK and PRK. *Exp. Eye Res.* 2003; 76:71-87.

[55] Ambrosio R Jr, Wilson S. LASIK vs LASEK vs PRK: advantages and indications. *Semin. Ophthalmol.* 2003; 18:2-30.

[56] Gauthier CA, Holden BA, Epstein D, et al. Role of epithelial hyperplasia in regression following photorefractive keratectomy. *Br. J. Ophthalmol.* 1996; 80:545-548.

[57] Lohmann CP, Guell JL. Regression after LASIK for the treatment of myopia: the role of the epithelium. *Semin. Ophthalmol.* 1998; 13:79-82.

[58] Wilson SE, He Y-G, Weng J, et al. Effect of epidermal growth factor, hepatocyte grwoth factor, and keratinocyte frowth factor on proliferation, motility and differentiation of human corneal epithelial cells. *Exp. Eye Res.* 1994; 59:665-78.

[59] Choi SY, Kim HY, Kim JY, et al. Two-year follow-up of eyes without topical corticosteroid treatment after photorefractive keratectomy (PRK). *Korean J. Ophthalmol.* 1998; 12:25-29.

[60] Corbett MC, O'Bart DP, Marshall J. Do topical corticosteroids have a role following excimer laser photorefractive keratectomy? *J. Refract. Surg.* 1995; 11:380-387.

[61] Gartry DS, Kerr Muir M, Marshall J. The effect of topical corticosteroids on refraction and corneal haze following excimer laser treatment of myopia: an update. A prospective, randomized, double-masked study. *Eye* 1993; 7:584-590.

[62] Vigo L, Scandola E, Carones F. Scraping and mitomycin C to treat haze and regression after photorefractive keratectomy for myopia. *J. Refract. Surg.* 2003; 19:449-454.

[63] Raviv T, Majmudar PA, Dennis RF, et al. Mitomycin-C for post-PRK corneal haze. *J. Cataract Refract. Surg.* 2000; 26:1105-1106.

[64] Carones F, Vigo L, Scandola E, et al. Evaluation of the prophylatice use of mitomycin-C to inhibit haze formation after photorefractive keratectomy. *J. Cataract Refract. Surg.* 2002; 28:2088-2095.

[65] Kasetsuwan N, Wu FM, Hsieh F, et al. Effect of topical ascorbic acid on free radical tissue damage and inflammatory cell influx in the corneal after excimer laser corneal surgery. *Arch. Ophthalmol.* 1999; 117:649-652.

[66] Stojanovic A, Ringvold A, Nitter T. Ascorbate prophylaxis for corneal haze after photorefractive keratectomy. *J. Refract. Surg.* 2003; 19:338-343.

[67] Anderson Penno E, Braun DA, Kamal A, et al. Topical thiotepa treatment for recurrent corneal haze after photorefractive keratectomy. *J. Cataract. Refract. Surg.* 2003; 29:1537-1542.

[68] Camellin M, Cimberle M. LASEK technique promising after 1 year of experience. *Ocul. Surg.* News 2000; 18:14-17.

[69] Lee JB, Seong GJ, Lee JH et al. Comparison of laser epithelial keratomileusis and photorefractive keratectomy for low to moderate myopia. *J. Cataract. Refract. Surg.* 2001; 27:565-570.

[70] Azar CT, Ang RT. Laser subepithelial keratomileusis: evolution of alcohol assisted flap surface ablation. *Int. Ophthalmol. Clin.* 2002; 42:89-97.

[71] Vinciguerra P, Camesasca FL. Butterfly laser epithelial keratomileusis for myopia. *J. Refract. Surg.* 2002; 18(3 Suppl):S371-S373.

[72] Samalonies LB. Gel-assisted LASEK. Eyeworld. February 2002. Available at: http://www.eyeworld.org/article.php?sid=2201. Accessed Feb 8, 2008.

[73] Chen CC, Change JH, Lee JB et al. Human corneal epithelial cell viability and morphology after dilute alcohol exposure. *Invest Oophthalmol. Vis. Sci.* 2002; 43:2593-602.

[74] Pallikaris IG, Katsanevaki VJ, Kalyvianaki MI, et al. Advances in subepithelial excimer refractive surgery techniques: Epi-LASIK. *Curr. Opin. Ophthalmol.* 2003; 14:207-212.

[75] Pallikaris IG, Katsanevaki VJ, Kalyvianaki MI, et al. Epi-LASIK: comparative histological evaluation of mechanical and alcohol-assisted epithelial separation. *J Cataract. Refract. Surg.*2003; 29;1496-1501.

[76] Hammond MD, Madigan WP, Bower KS. Refractive Surgery in the US Army: 2000 – 2003. *Ophthalmology* 2005 Feb;112:184-190.)

[77] Pop M, Payette Y. Photorefractive keratectomy versus laser in situ keratomileusis. *Ophthalmol.* 2000; 107:251-257.

[78] El Danasoury MC, Maghraby AE, Elyce SD et al. Comparison of photorefractive keratectomy with excimer laser in situ keratomileusis in correcting low myopia (from -2.00 to -5.50 diopters). A randomized study. *Ophthalmol.* 1999; 106:411-421.

[79] Ghadfan F, Al;Rajhi A, Wagoner MD. Laser in situ keratomileusis versus surface ablation: Visual outcomes and complications. *J. Cataract refract. Surg.* 2007; 33:2041-2048.

[80] Jabbur NS. Endothelial cell studies in patients after photorefractive keratectomy for hyperopia. *J. Refract. Surg*. 2003; 19:142-148.

[81] Diakonis VF, Pallikaris A, Kymionis GD, et al. Alterations in endothelial cell density after photorefractive keratectomy with adjuvant mitomycin. *Am. J. Ophthalmol.* 2007; 144:99-103.

[82] Shah S, Sebai Sarhan AR, Doyle SJ, et al. The epithelial flap for photorefractive keratectomy. *Br. J. Ophthalmol.* 2001; 85:393-396.

[83] Gamaly TO, El Danasoury A, El Maghraby A. A prospective, randomized, contralateral eye comparison of epithelial laser in situ keratomileusis and photorefractive keratectomy in eyes prone to haze. *J. Refract. Surg.* 2007; 23(Suppl):S1015-S1020

In: Laser Keratectomy: Approaches, Complications...
Author: Luis W. Schröder and Felix J. Walter
ISBN 978-1-60456-863-9


*Chapter VI*

# Optimized Profiles for "Aberration-Free" Refractive Surgery

***Diego de Ortueta*[1] *, Thomas Magnago*[2] *and Samuel Arba-Mosquera*[2]**
[1] Augenzentrum Recklinghausen, Germany
[2] Schwind eye-tech-solutions GmbH,
Kleinhostheim, Germany

## 1. Perspective of Aberration-Free Profiles

The first goal of a laser treatment for refractive surgery is to balance the refractive defects of an eye. The optical quality of an eye is significantly determined through low and high order aberrations. These always define an optical error, regardless of whether they are corneal or ocular aberrations.

We have low order aberrations as sphere and cylinder and high order aberrations such coma, spherical aberration, trefoil or pentafoil. It can occur, and actually, it is often the case, that the best approach for planning and ablation is a sophisticated pattern, which can still be described simply in terms of sphere, cylinder, and orientation (axis). Studies[1,2] of untreated eyes show that patients with above-average visual acuity (somehow individuals achieving supervision) can have moderate amounts of high-order aberrations. It was also observed that the individuals with the least amount of aberrations were not necessarily the ones scoring the highest visual acuities. In these studies, performed among populations with supernormal vision, no direct relationship between these high-order aberrations and visual performance of untreated eyes could be determined. Moreover, because the brain adjusts to aberrations through the help of neural compensation[3], and these aberrations are in the experience of the patient as normal, it is not always advantageous to remove all aberrations through laser correction. There is some plasticity[4] of the neural system so that distortions in the visual field are corrected, but as patients are viewing the world through their own wave aberration they will reject corrections which are too large from their "normal" experience. With aberration-free patterns we tailor the eye's subjective sphero-cylindrical refractive error, different of the term wavefront guided where the high order aberrations are also corrected.

Some studies on treated eyes found that wavefront guided treatments induce less aberration than conventional profiles, but they are not actually reducing the preoperative aberrations, indeed they created new ones[5,6].

In this context an „Aberration-Free“ treatment is optimum for patients whose sight is not affected by existing high-order aberrations and for those who – only corrected with glasses - possess a visual acuity of 1.0 or better. With this treatment, the (pre-operative) high-order aberrations remain unchanged. The advantage is that the patient retains the habitual sight impression ("visual print") at best focus and the brain requires no learning phase to deal with otherwise added bothersome changes. The ideal profile „Aberration-Free“ means that the laser treatment, with a highly sophisticated pattern is delivered in such way that only spherical and/or cylindrical refractive values are corrected. No optical high-order aberrations are changed nor additional aberrations induced that could reduce vision sharpness and contrast, as opposed to classical, Munnerlyn-based[7] treatments and a number of aspheric methods used in the market that induce aberrations.. Thus, the pre-operative and post-operative high order aberrations are identical. So that we are treating the eye in a neutral way. The goal is to correct the manifest refraction without inducing or changing the aberrations of the eye.

If the diagnostically assessed high-order aberrations impair the visual performance, they should be corrected. In those cases we recommend wavefront-guided treatments[8] as the right choice, when corneal[9,10] and/or ocular wavefront data[11] can be included. We should plan the most optimum ablation pattern specifically for each individual eye based on its anamnesis, diagnosis, and visual demands and allow even more individual, patient-oriented treatment.

## 2. Advantages of Aberration-Free Profile

Let us make some historical review of the different profile definitions used since the beginning of Laser refractive surgery.

Laser corneal refractive surgery is based on the use of a Laser (typically an excimer one) to change the corneal curvature to compensate for refractive errors of the eye[12]. It has become the most successful technique, mainly due to the submicron precision and the high repeatability of the ablation of the cornea accompanied by minimal side effects[13].

„Classical approaches“ for sphero-cylindrical correction include:

*Munnerlyn based profiles*: where the profile is calculated as the difference of two spheres:

$$z=\left(R_2-\sqrt{R_2^2-r^2}\right)-\left(R-\sqrt{R^2-r^2}\right) \qquad \frac{(n-1)}{R_2}=\frac{(n-1)}{R}+D$$

where, the z is the ablation depth, r is the radial distance to the ablation centre, and $R_2$ is predicted postoperative radius of curvature, R is the preoperative radius of curvature, n the refractive index of the cornea, and D the amount of dioptres to be corrected.

Munnerlyn based profiles induce aberrations, with a theoretical post-operative increase of "prolateness" after myopic treatments[14]:

- Q-value becomes more negative after myopic treatments, and more positive after hyperopic ones
- Induced aberrations depend on the pre-operative keratometries
- Induced aberrations depend on the dioptric power change

The Munnerlyn profile assumes that if epithelium is removed and a portion of stroma ablated, the epithelium will regrow with a uniform thickness and produce a new corneal curvature determined by the new curvature of the stroma.

*Parabolic based profiles:* where the profile is calculated as a parabola:

$$z = \frac{Dr^2}{2(n-1)}$$

where, the z is the ablation depth, r is the radial distance to the ablation centre, n the refractive index of the cornea, and D the amount of dioptres to be corrected.

Parabolic based profiles induce aberrations, with a theoretical post-operative decrease of "prolateness" after myopic treatments[14]:

- Q-value becomes more positive after myopic treatments, and more negative after hyperopic ones
- Induced aberrations depend on the pre-operative keratometries
- Induced aberrations depend on the dioptric power change

One of the most significant side effects in laser corneal refractive surgery with classical approaches is the induction of spherical aberration[15] which causes halos and reduced contrast sensitivity[16], resulting in deviations from the optimal corneal line-shape post-operatively. Some reasons can be argumented to explain, at least in part, these deviations:

1) Profile definitions based on improper physical approaches (the theoretical models used to develop the profiles might have been too simple)[17]
2) None or improper methods for balancing the loss of ablation efficiency due to non-normal incidence of the surgical beam[18,19,20,21].
3) Biomechanical reactions of the cornea. There are some biological response of the cornea after laser ablation[22].

To avoid the induction of aberrations, the so-called "customised" treatments were developed. Customisation of the ablation is possible either using wavefront measurements of the whole eye[23] (obtained, e.g., by Hartman-Shack wavefront sensors[24]) or by using corneal topography[25] or derived wavefront analyses[26]. In this case the low and high order aberrations are treated. With these patterns it was expected to create supervision, as image quality should be improved[27]. If we analyze the results of the different ablation pattern we can see that in some cases they created "supervison" but in reality they are creating less aberrations as the conventional classical profiles but not decreasing the preoperatively high order aberrations[28].

The advantages of the "Aberration-Free" ablation profiles vs. classical profiles are, for instance: aspherical profiles to balance the induction of spherical aberration (optimized asphericity controlling the postoperative corneal asphericity) in a way that the HOA are preserved. They provide K-reading compensation, which considers the change in spot geometry and reflection losses of ablation efficiency.

## 3. The Aberration-Free Pattern of SCHWIND

The SCHWIND system works with two laser platforms the AMARIS and the ESIRIS. Both are flying spot laser with a small beam profile. The ESIRIS works with a repetition rate of 200 Hz and a spot diameter of 0.8 mm (FWHM)[29,30]. The compensations of the lateral eye movements are done with a 330 Hz Eye-Tracker[31] with 5-ms latency period[32] which still is one of the fastest trackers even after years. Based on this experience the AMARIS is the successor and combines the technology of static and dynamic cyclotorsion[33,34,35], limbus tracking and compensation of the eye's rolling movement[36] under an eye-tracker which works with 1050 Hz and 3-ms latency period. The laser itself provides true 500 Hz at a spot diameter of 0.54 mm (FWHM) at two different fluence levels. One higher lever of fluence for quickness and another lower level for preciseness. Altogether this leads to a treatment time of less than 2.5 s per myopic diopter.

SCHWIND ORK-CAM (Optimized Refractive Keratectomy Custom Ablation Manager) is a software developed to import, visualise, and analyse diagnostic data of the eye (manifest refraction, corneal wavefront, or ocular wavefront data). It calculates the highly precise aspheric ablation profiles for sphero-cylindric aberration-free treatment as well as for wavefront-guided corrections. An individual ablation volume will be exported to the SCHWIND AMARIS / ESIRIS laser system for the correction of refractive errors.

Based on diagnostic data the ORK-CAM software, following advanced algorithms, is capable to integrate ocular wavefront data or topography based corneal wavefront data into the refractive treatment procedure in order to achieve optimum refractive outcomes and visual qualities[37,38,39,40].

The Aberration-Free ablation profile itself, which is the matter of this section, is based on statistical investigation about the optimal content of certain high order aberrations on vision. Physically a clear correlation between an aspheric corneal line-shape function and high order spherical aberration terms exist[41]. Hence, it is possible generate an asphere out of given spherocylindical correction data using a well-defined and certain amount of high order aberrations. In the CAM software an optimized outcome (aberration-free = optimized asphericity) is thus aspired.

With both of the treatment methods, the „Aberration-Free" as well as the „Wavefront-Guided" treatment, the aspherical ablation profile is employed. The aspherical ablation profiles of the SCHWIND ORK-CAM software module ensure that induced aberrations through biomechanical influences are compensated. Such influences include microkeratome cut, tissue removal of the cornea, as well as varying energy losses depending on the corneal curvature during laser correction.

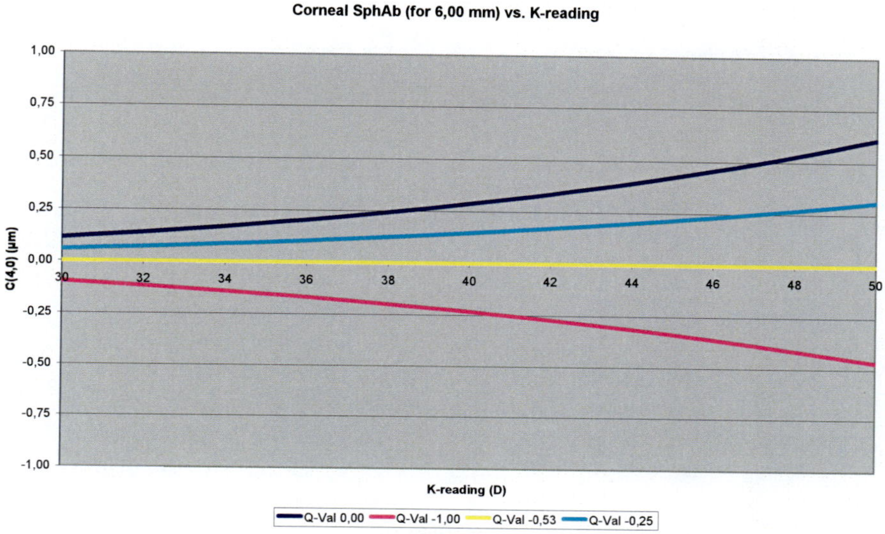


Figure 1. Corneal Spherical Aberration vs. Keratometry for 4 different representative anterior corneal surface models: Spherical corneal model (in dark blue), Parabolic corneal model (in purple), "Free-of-aberrations" corneal model (in yellow) and Balanced corneal model (in light blue).

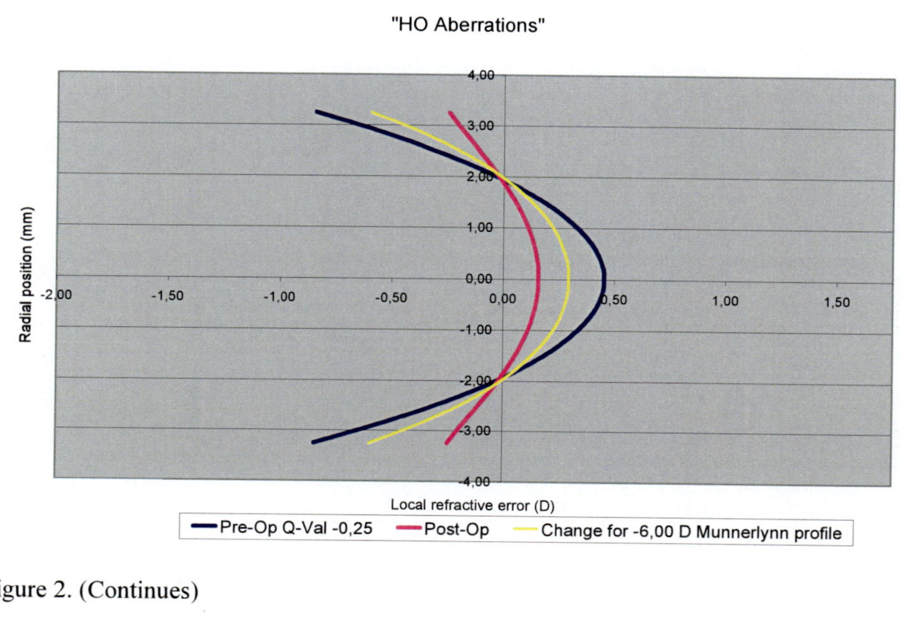


Figure 2. (Continues)

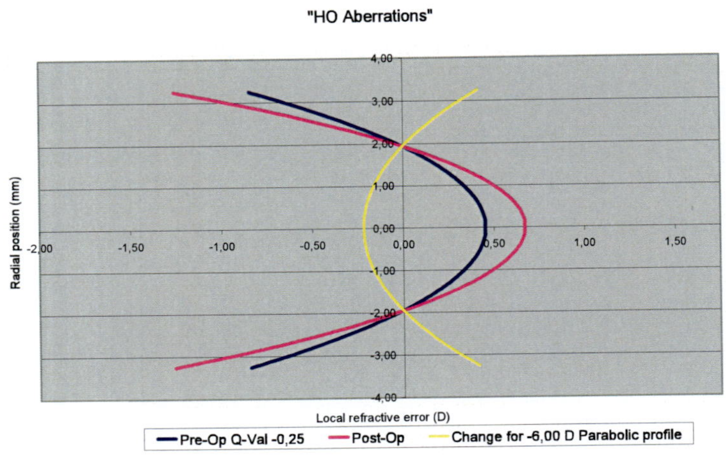


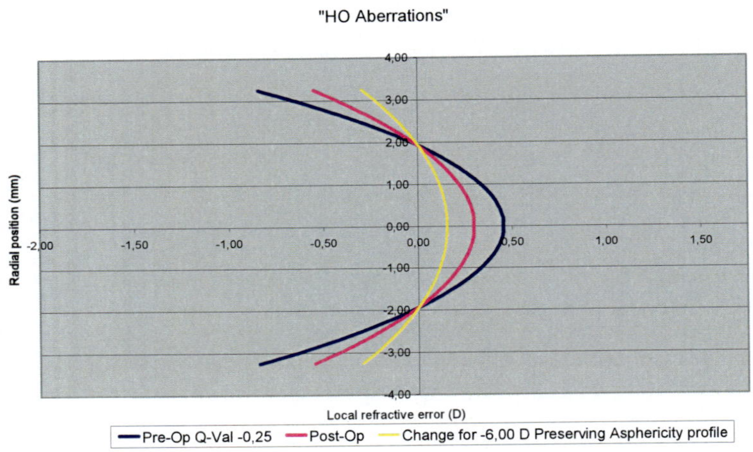


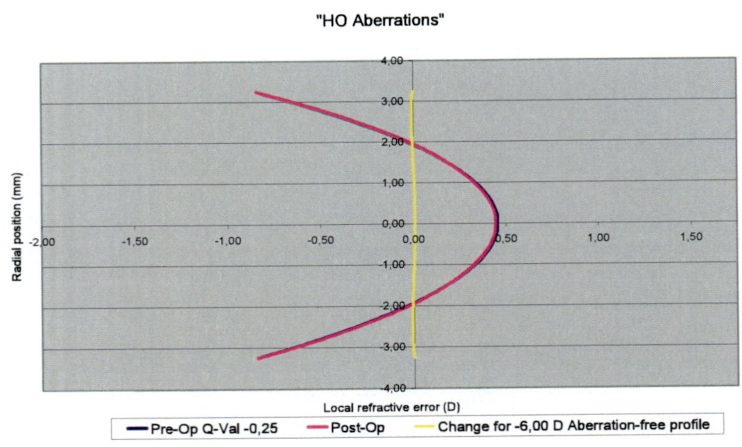


Figure 2. Induced Corneal Spherical Aberration for -6.00 D at 6.50 mm for a balanced corneal model, for 4 different ablation profiles: Munnerlyn based profiles, Parabolic based profiles, Asphericity preserving profiles, Aberration-free profiles. Notice the pre-op aberrated status (in blue), the post-op aberrated status (in purple), and the induced aberrations (in yellow)

The Aberration free approach for sphero-cylindrical correction includes compensations for many possible sources of aberrations after LASER refractive procedures[42] as: biomechanical reactions due to the flap cu[43,44], wrong defined "optimized" line-shapes, wrong defined blending zones, loss of ablation efficiency considerations, pattern off-centrations, spot size limitations[45,46], active Eye-Tracking capabilities[47,48,49], biomechanical reactions due to the ablation process itself[50].

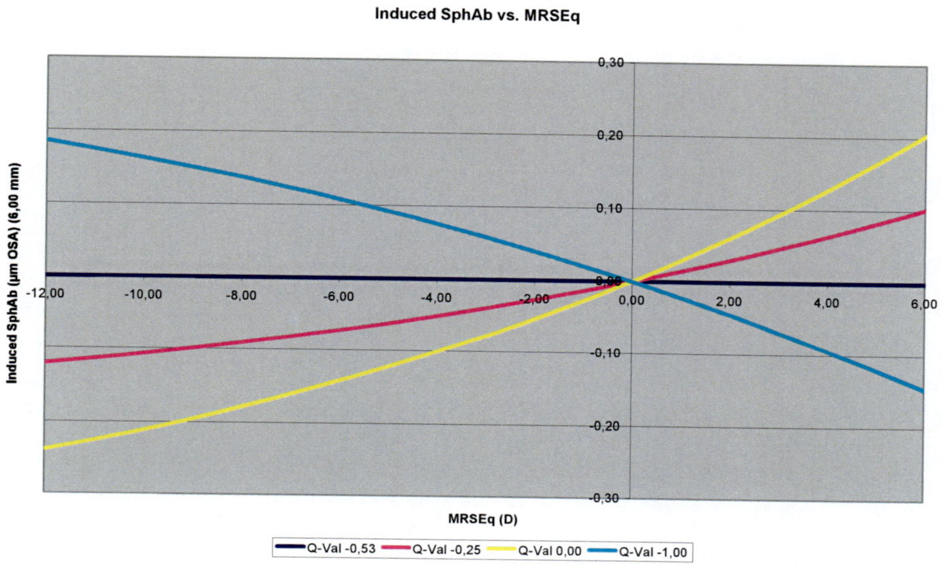


Figure 3. Induced Corneal Spherical Aberration vs. Refractive correction for 4 different representative ablation profile definitions: Aberration-Free profiles (in dark blue), Asphericity preserving profiles (in purple), Munnerlyn based profiles (in yellow) and Parabolic based profiles (in light blue)

*Aberration-Free based profiles*: To compensate for as many of those sources of aberrations as possible, in a way as efficient as possible, SCHWIND eye-tech-solutions has developed Aberration-Free based profiles: where the profile balances the effects on the Wavefront Aberration:

$$HOWFAb_{Post}(\rho,\theta) = HOWFAb_{Pre}(\rho,\theta) \quad \forall \rho,\theta \in OZ$$
$$\Delta HOWFAb(\rho,\theta) = 0 \quad \forall \rho,\theta \in OZ$$

Aberration-free profiles DO NOT induce aberrations, with a theoretical post-operative decrease of "prolateness":

- Q-value becomes more positive after myopic treatments, and more negative after hyperopic ones
- NO induced aberrations, INDEPENDENT on the pre-operative keratometries
- NO induced aberrations, INDEPENDENT on the dioptric change

- NO induced aberrations, INDEPENDENT on the Asphericity
- Aberration-free profiles DO NOT induce aberrations
- SCHWIND's approach will provide normal eyes with the best quality of vision, without affecting their perception of the World.
- They are different from Munnerlyn based profiles
- They are different from Parabolic based profiles
- They are different from Asphericity based profiles
- They must be, as well, the base-line for Customised profiles

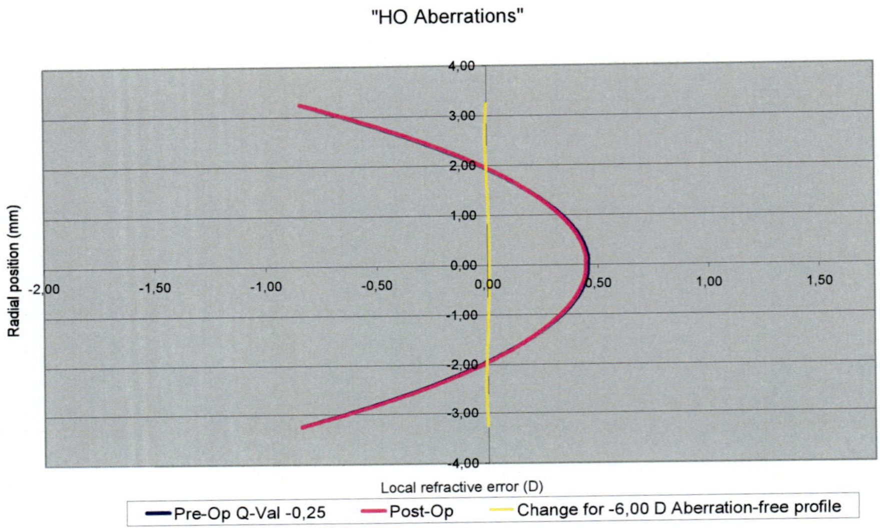


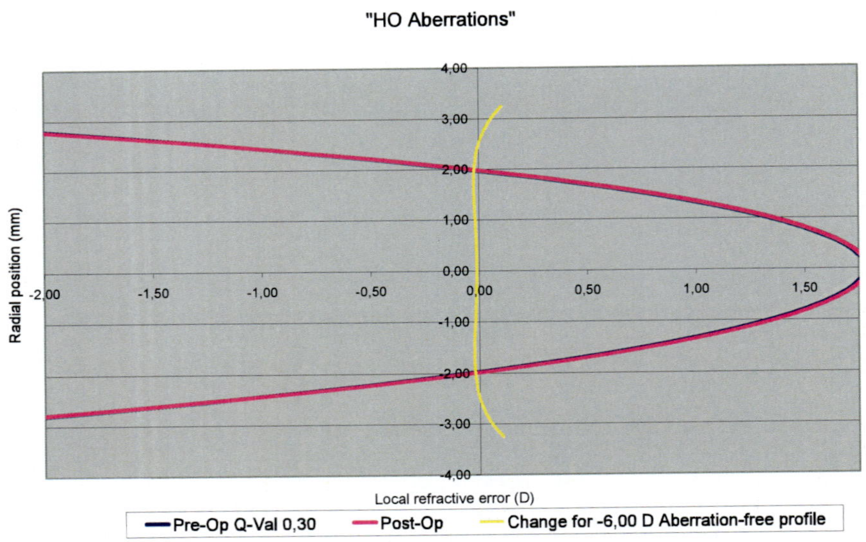


Figure 4. (Continues)

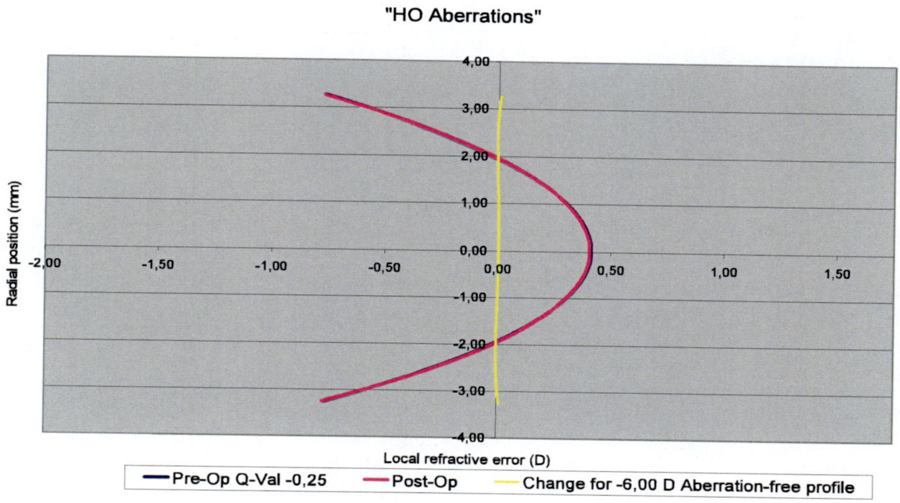


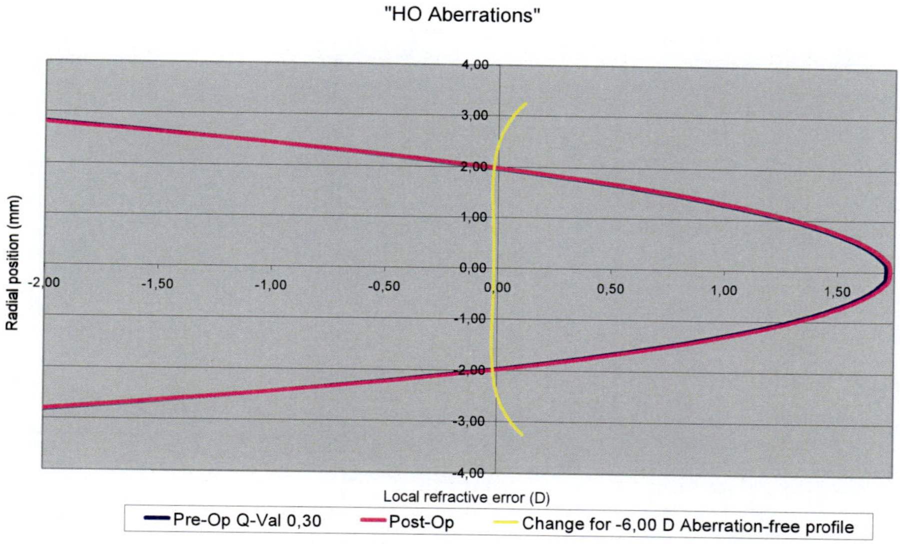


Figure 4. Induced Spherical Aberration using SCHWIND Aberration-Free profiles for -6.00 D at 6.50 mm for 2 anterior corneal surfaces (in columns): 7.87 mm, Q -0.25; and 7.03 mm, Q +0.30; and for 2 posterior corneal surfaces and pachymetries (in rows): 525 µm central pachymetry, 775 µm peripheral pachymetry at 5 mm radial distance; and 550 µm central pachymetry, 550 µm peripheral pachymetry at 5 mm radial distance. Notice the pre-op aberrated status (in blue), the post-op aberrated status (in purple), and the induced aberrations (in yellow).

Schwind CAM Aberration-free profiles balance other sources of aberration, reducing the refractive power by means of modulating the corneal radii of curvature according to the planned refractive correction but without introducing optical wavefront aberrations ($\Delta WFE_{HO}$=0), resulting in no induction of High Order Aberrations. The patients will maintain the same level of High Order aberrations as pre-operative. In particular, no Spherical aberration (related to halos) is induced, no coma (related with double images) is induced, and no trefoil is induced, providing a better visual quality post-operative.

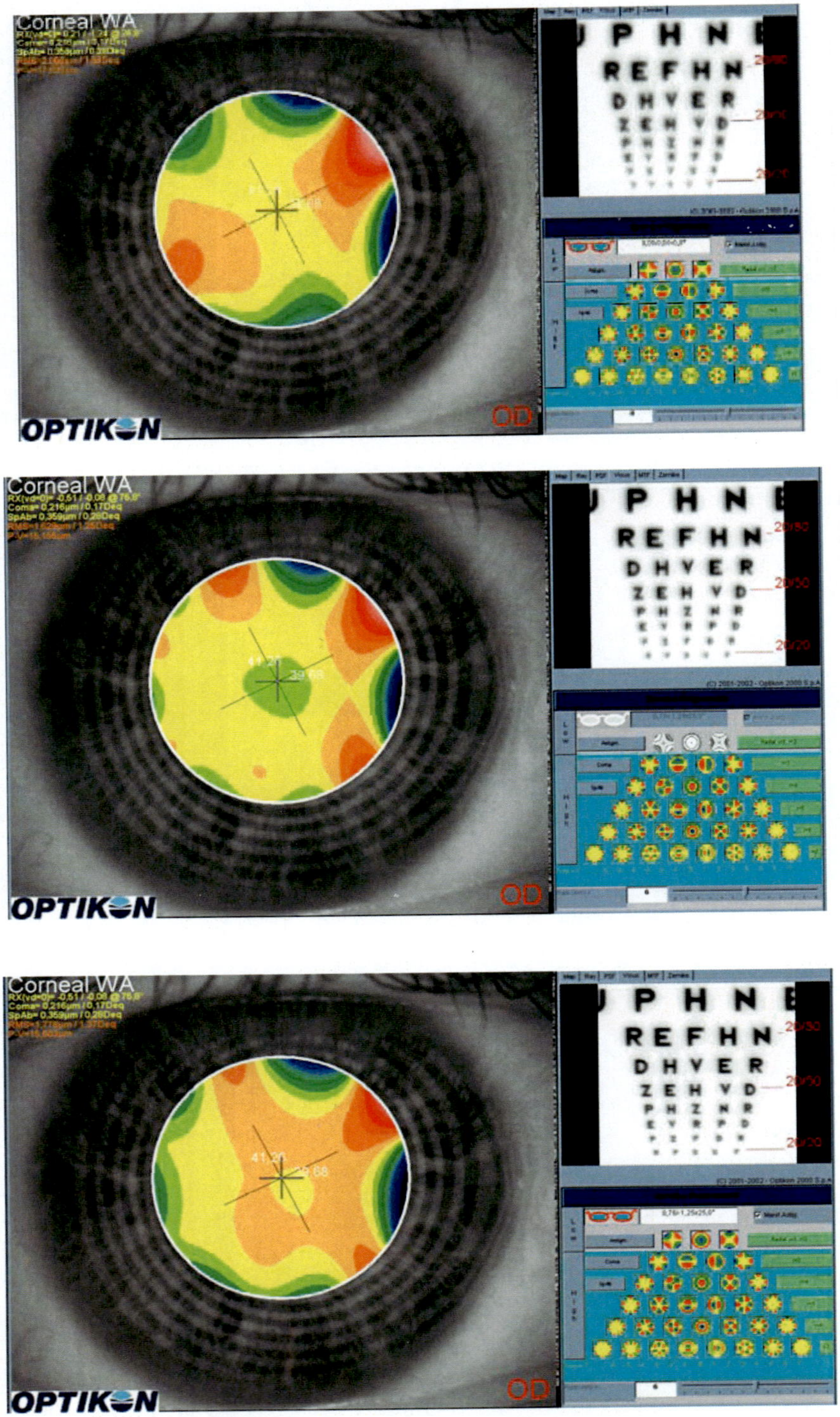


Figure 5. Wavefront aberration and simulated visus for different treatment strategies: preoperative status (top), simulation after low orders correction (middle), simulation after Aberration-Free correction (bottom). Notice the better visual quality after Aberraion-Free correction

Figure 5 shows the improvement and the benefit of the aberration-free strategy which considers the combined effect of the refraction (lower order aberration) and the high order aberrations. The software creates an aspherical ablation profile to optimize the corneal shape. Using „Aberration-free" profiles, ablations are optimized to induce no change in Wavefront aberration (within Optical Zone) other than Sphere and Cylinder components, leaving all existing high order aberrations (HOA) unchanged because the best corrected visual acuity, in this patient, has been unaffected by the pre-existing aberrations. Thus to compensate for the aberrations induction observed with other types of profile definitions[51].

Such a profile fulfils the "aberration-free" statement for a profile:

$$HOWFAb_{Post}(\rho,\theta) = HOWFAb_{\mathrm{Pre}}(\rho,\theta) \quad \forall \rho,\theta \in OZ$$
$$\Delta HOWFAb(\rho,\theta) = 0 \qquad \forall \rho,\theta \in OZ$$

where HOWFAb means High Order Wavefront Aberration.

Meaning that, the Wavefront aberration (within Optical Zone) after surgery equals the Wavefront aberration (within Optical Zone) prior to the surgery after balancing Sphere and Cylinder components. In other words, there is no induced change in Wavefront aberration (within Optical Zone) other than Sphere and Cylinder components. Thus, balancing the effects on the Wavefront aberration, and providing normal eyes with the best quality of vision, without affecting their perception of the World ("visual print").

We want to clarify that this „aberration-free" profile definition is definitely different from an aspherical profile designed to preserve corneal asphericity, where the goal is described in terms of elevation and shape parameters, rather than in terms of wavefront aberration.

*Aspherical based profiles*: where the profile is calculated as the difference of two aspheres[52]:

$$z = \frac{R_2}{Q_2+1}\left(1-\sqrt{1-(Q_2+1)\left(\frac{r}{R_2}\right)^2}\right) - \frac{R}{Q+1}\left(1-\sqrt{1-(Q+1)\left(\frac{r}{R}\right)^2}\right) \qquad \frac{(n-1)}{R_2} = \frac{(n-1)}{R} + D$$

Asphericity based profiles induce aberrations, with a theoretical post-operative preservation or modulation of "prolateness"[53]:

- Q-value remains stable or reaches a predefined level after myopic or hyperopic treatments
- Induced aberrations depend on the pre-operative keratometries
- Induced aberrations depend on the dioptric power change
- Example correction of asphericity based myopia:
- Reduction of refractive power by means of flattening the corneal radius of curvature but preserving the prolate corneal line shape (Q=-0.25)
- Issues for Asphericity Optimisation:

- The Asphericity is an abstract value, it is not independent. It is only a concept that related to the paraxial radius of curvature represents a good approximation of the corneal surface[54]
- The paraxial radius of curvature and the asphericity do not represent optical errors, but absolute elevation
- Forcing the post-operative asphericity to remain unchanged is, somehow, like forcing the paraxial radius of curvature to remain unchanged
- Forcing the post-operative asphericity to remain unchanged induces aberrations (Spherical Aberration and High-Order Astigmatism)
- By itself does not cover corneal biomechanics

Another problem using Q-factor customised ablation profiles is the severe difficulties to determine the Q-factor to be targeted. The average asphericity of the human cornea is about -0.28[55]. Nevertheless, there are persons with Q -0.25 and poor vision, and others with Q +0.25 and supervision. Despite of some remarkable theoretical works[56,57,58], there is no prove that more negative Q-factors provide better visual quality, or that an absolute optimum exists[59].

Because "aberration-free" profile as defined does not require preserving corneal asphericity, we are, somehow, customising the target Q-Value for each single treatment and controlling, therefore, the postoperative asphericity.

Let us now have a closer look at the specific characteristics offered in the Schwind CAM ablation planner.

The ORK-CAM software provides different levels of detail:

- *Aspherical treatments*: Based on Aberration-Free aspherical profiles, where only the spherical and cylindrical intended refractive change is needed together with the corneal keratometries.
- *Corneal Wavefront treatments*: Based on Corneal Ray Tracing linked to the SCHWIND Corneal Wavefront Analyzer: OPTIKON Keratron Scout/Bridge and CSO Eye-Top
- *Ocular wavefront treatments:* Based on Hartmann-Shack Sensing linked o the SCHWIND Ocular Wavefront Analyzer
- General optimum in non-wavefront-driven refractive surgery is to balance the effects on the Wavefront aberration, and, to provide normal eyes with the best quality of vision, without affecting their perception of the world:
- Aberration-Free treatments have the advantage of saving tissue, time and due to their relative simplicity offer a very high predictability
- Corneal Wavefront treatments have the advantage of being independent from accommodation effects or light/pupil conditions
- Ocular Wavefront treatments have the advantage of being based on Objective Refraction of the complete optical system of the human eye
- SCHWIND ORK-CAM introduces a new sophisticated algorithm establishing new standards in laser corneal refractive surgery:
- Aspheric ablation profiles result in an optimized post-operative Q-value

- Planning of treatments, depending on the level of detail asked for, based only on sphero-cylindrical input as well as on imported corneal wavefront or ocular wavefront data
- Advanced algorithms in order to achieve optimum refractive outcomes and visual qualities
- Extremely smooth surfaces and "mild" ablation by using a defined pulse sorting algorithm

Key factors in the ORK-CAM profiles:

- Without nomogram adjustments, it provides different ablation ratios for PRK/LASEK or LASIK treatments
- Multi-Dynamic Transition zone
- The 3-dimensional shape of the Transition Zone are of great importance in ablation pattern algorithms design because they smooth the ablated area towards the non-treated cornea.
- 3+ Aspherical Dimensions
- Enhanced Energy Correction to compensate the loss of ablation efficiency

Energy Correction algorithms have been refined including the influence coming from flying-spot technology where the interspot spacing is small compared to the spot width and multiple spots overlap each other contributing to the ablation at each corneal location

## Different Ablation Ratios for PRK/LASEK or LASIK Treatments

It has been empirically observed that the same ablation profile results in different actual ablations when applied to the outer surface of the anterior cornea (PRK) or to the corneal stroma (LASIK):

Possible reasons for these different ablation ratios for PRK and LASIK can be:

- Different LASER-Tissue interaction properties (Corneal irradiance threshold and absorption coefficient, different density or type of the collagen fibers)[61]

Corneal irradiance threshold is not uniquely defined ranging from 40 to 60 mJ/cm$^2$
Corneal absorption coefficient is also not uniquely defined ranging from 3.33 to 3.99 m$^{-1}$

- Different corneal refractive indexes (cornea structured in layers)

Corneal refractive index[62] is, as well, not uniquely defined ranging from 1.332 to 1.378

To account for this effect, SCHWIND eye-tech-solutions has implemented an Ablative spot volume differently modelised for PRK/LASEK and LASIK treatments, resulting in less need for nomograms.

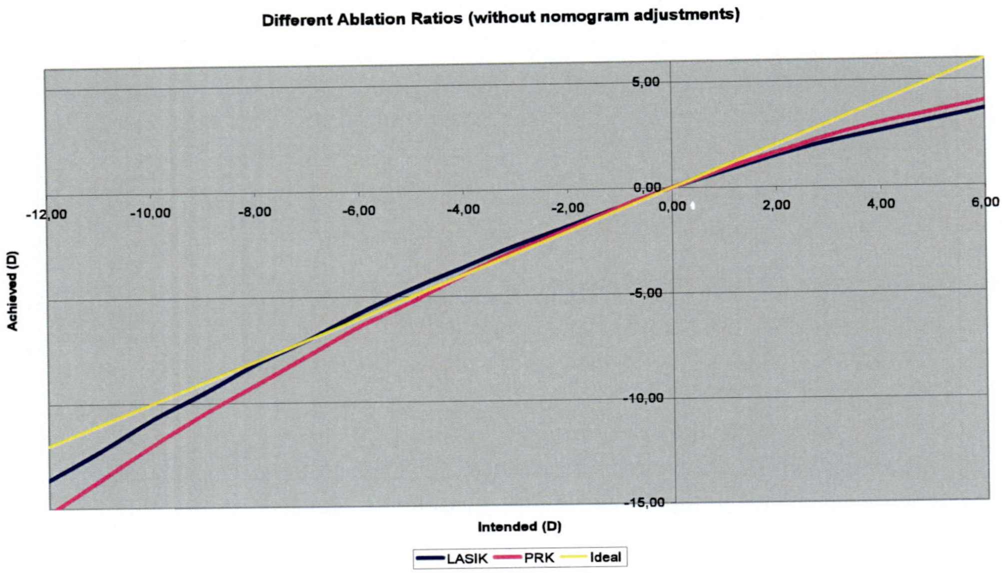


Figure 6. Intended vs. achieved correction using classical profiles for different treatment strategies: LASIK (in blue), PRK (in purple), reference ideal 1:1 line (in yellow). Notice that PRK treatments (historically the first ones) were relatively accurate for low to moderate myopic corrections, overcorrected for high myopic corrections and undercorrected for hyperopic corrections, whereas LASIK treatments were undercorrected for low myopic corrections, relatively accurate for moderate myopic corrections, slightly overcorrected for high myopic corrections and undercorrected for hyperopic corrections[60]

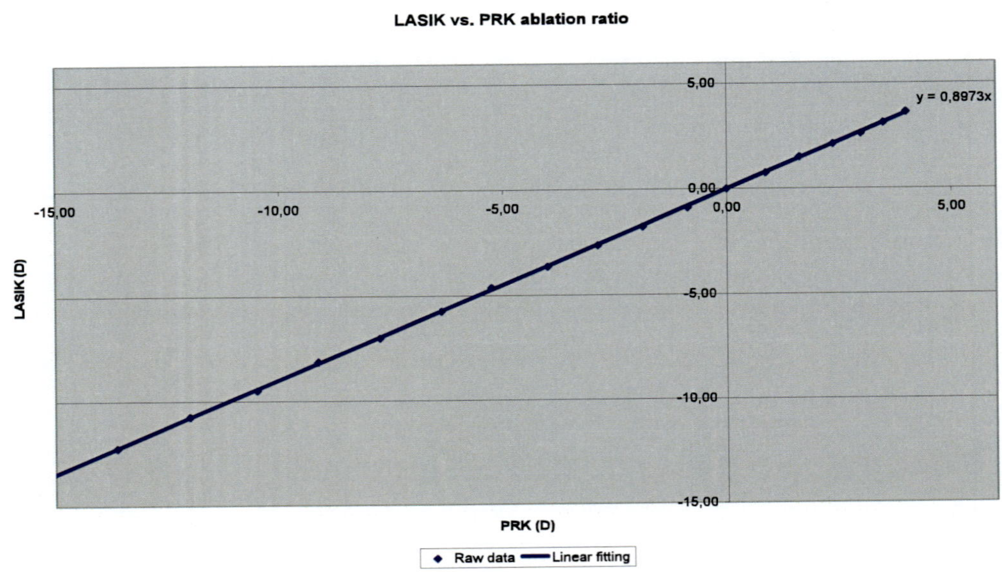


Figure 7. Relative LASIK vs. PRK achieved corrections. Notice the clear LASIK undercorrection when using PRK nomogram adjustments.

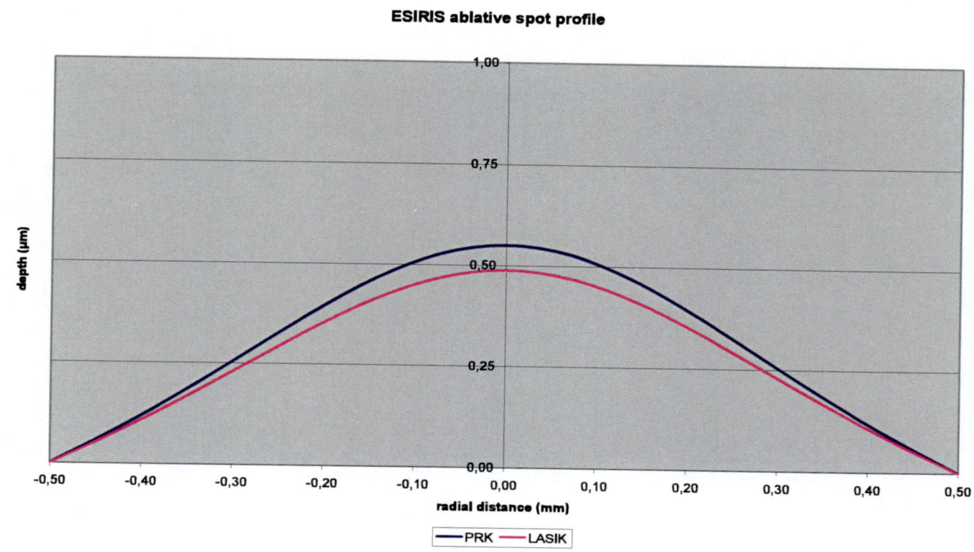


Figure 8. Unique Schwind different ablative spot profiles for surface (PRK) (in blue) and stromal (LASIK) (in purple) tissues. Notice that the smaller the spot, the more the number of pulses compensating for the relative undercorrection of stromal vs. surface ablation.

## Multi-Dynamic Transition Zone

Blending/Transition Zones are of great importance in ablation pattern algorithms design because they smooth the ablated area towards the non-treated cornea[63]. Blending/Transition Zones are, somehow, responsible of providing the actual functional Optical Zone[64]. Important amount of induced Coma, Spherical Aberration, and High Order Astigmatism aberrations are coming from eye tilts, decentration and "edge" effects[65], the strong local curvature change from Optical to Transition zones and from Transition Zone to the non-treated corneal tissue. It is necessary to emphasise the use of huge Optical Zones (trying to cover the scotopic pupil size plus some tolerance for possible decentrations), and well-defined smooth Transition Zones. But it does not mean that the huger the Transition Zone, the better the smoothing effect (thus the refractive result)

SCHWIND eye-tech-solutions has introduced a Transition Zone definition based on Slope Transition Factors leading to no unnecessary extra ablation for hyperopic treatments, and the "Transition Factors" are balanced between the edge of the Optical Zone and the edge of the Total Ablation Zone.

This Transition Zone definition minimises the red rings (after myopic corrections, blue rings after hyperopic corrections) observed at the edges of the Optical Zone in the topography (curvature map), and it enhances the effective functional Optical Zone.

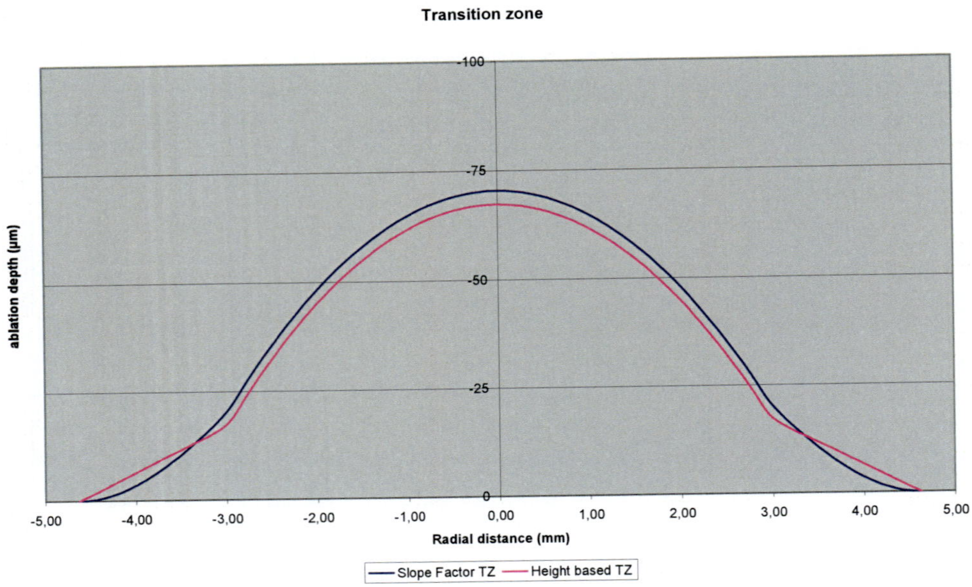


Figure 9. Slope factor Transition Zone (in blue) vs. Height based Transition Zone (in purple) for a myopic correction. Notice that height based Transition Zone produce a strong curvature change at the edge of the Optical Zone, opposed to a better smoothing effect of the Slope based Transition Zone.

Finally, Transition Zone is automatically determined by the software in a multifactorial dynamic way depending on:

- Refraction (-3D get a different Transition Zone than -6D)
- Type of refraction (myopia differs from hyperopia)
- Technique (LASIK differs from PRK and LASEK)
- Detail level (aspherical differs from customised)
- Optical Zone (the Transition Zone is different for 4 mm Optical Zone or for 7 mm Optical Zone).

With this approach, surgeons do not need to worry about the selection of the optimal necessary transition zone, which is then standardised (same treatment will get exactly same Transition Zone), and this Transition Zone represents the minimal tissue and time required for that correction to be optimally ablated.

Meaning of the "3+ Aspherical Dimensions" in the ORK-CAM profiles:

- 1st Aspherical Dimension: The profile mainly compensates for the Spherical Aberration induced by the Transition Zone (True Optical Zones)
- 2nd Aspherical Dimension: The profile compensates for the Spherical Aberration induced by the ablation itself (corneal biomechanics related to removal of corneal tissue and to post-operative intraocular pressure)
- 3rd Aspherical Dimension: The LASIK profile compensates for the Spherical Aberration induced by the flap cut itself (corneal biomechanics)

- Plus: The profile compensates for the Loss of ablation efficiency produced by the corneal curvature when ablating at non-normal incidence.

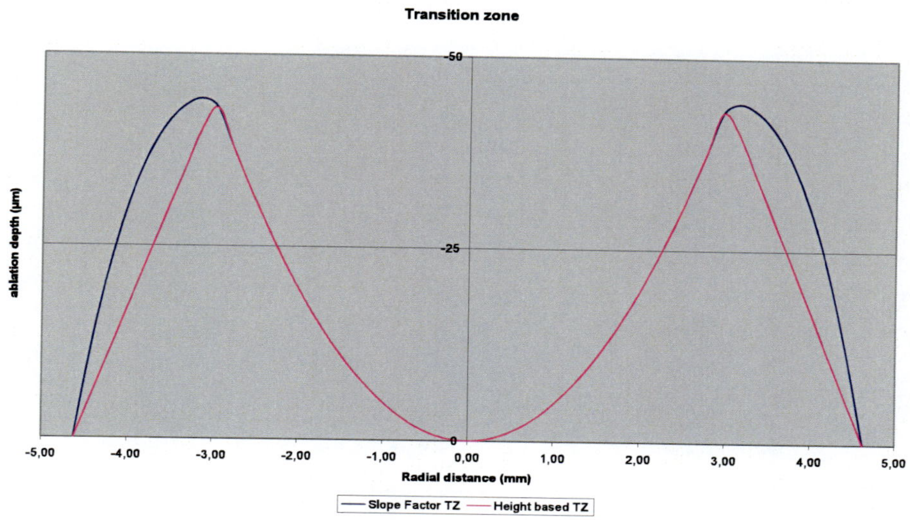


Figure 10. Slope factor Transition Zone (in blue) vs. Height based Transition Zone (in purple) for a hyperopic correction. Notice that height based Transition Zone produce a very steep curvature change at the edge of the Optical Zone, whereas slope based Transition Zone ablates deeper beyond the Optical Zone boundaries but with decreasing slope smoothing out the ablation edges.

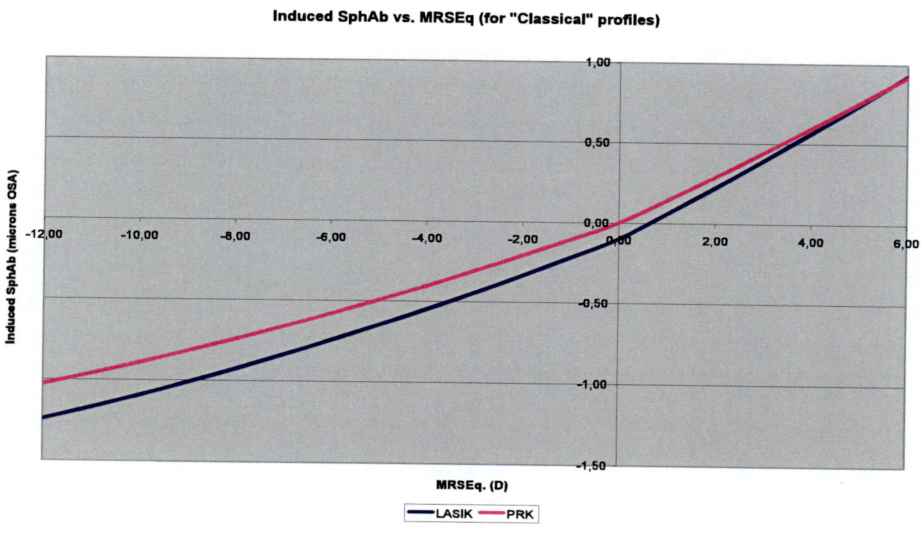


Figure 11. Induced Spherical aberration vs. achieved correction using classical profiles for different treatment strategies: LASIK (in blue), PRK (in purple). Notice that LASIK induced Spherical aberration does not go across the origin, representing the isolated effect due to the flap cut treatments. Notice as well that the induced Spherical aberration was more pronounced for hyperopic treatments than for myopic ones[66]

## Enhanced Energy Correction to Compensate the Loss of Ablation Efficiency

K-readings are used to account for the energy correction by means of the local curvature change and related local energy lost at different spot positions across the ablation area (especially interesting for pathological corneas).

The standard model used for loss of ablation efficiency (when included in the systems) considers the actual material removed at any point depending only on the shots targeting this point. A refined model including the influence coming from flying-spot technology, in which the interspot spacing is small compared to the spot width and multiple spots overlap each other contributing to the ablation at each corneal location, is provided at the CAM software, including the actual incidence angle for the beam at any single aspherical corneal location including astigmatism, as well as, the progressive effect of the ablation procedure where the corneal radii are changing throughout the treatment.

The beam is reduced due to the loss of reflected energy, but, at the same time, it is expanded due to the angular projection.

## Requirements to Gain Optimal Laser Shot Distribution

Both the AMARIS and the ESIRIS systems are flying-spot lasers using randomised spot distribution to minimise thermal effects.

The AMARIS laser system works at a repetition rate of 500 Hz, produces a spot size of 0.54 mm (full width at half maximum (FWHM)) with a superGaussian ablative spot profile. High-speed eye-tracking with 1050 Hz acquisition rate is accomplished with 3-ms latency period.

The ESIRIS laser system works at a repetition rate of 200 Hz and produces a spot size of 0.8 mm (FWHM) with a paraGaussian ablative spot profile. Eye-Tracking is accomplished with 330 Hz acquisition rate and 5 ms latency time.

The gained ablation volume has to be applied onto the cornea by thousands of single laser shots at different but partly repeated corneal positions, because the ablated volume of a single spot is much smaller than the ablation volume.

SCHWIND eye-tech-solutions has introduced as well some innovations concerning ablation shot file (sequences of pulses needed to carry out a refractive procedure) generation, in order to optimally remove the tissue corresponding to these state-of-the-art treatments including:

- "Aberration-Free" aspheric lens design
- Enhanced energy correction
- laser spot profile modulation
- Improved spot overlap matrix
- Statistical laser spot sorting algorithm

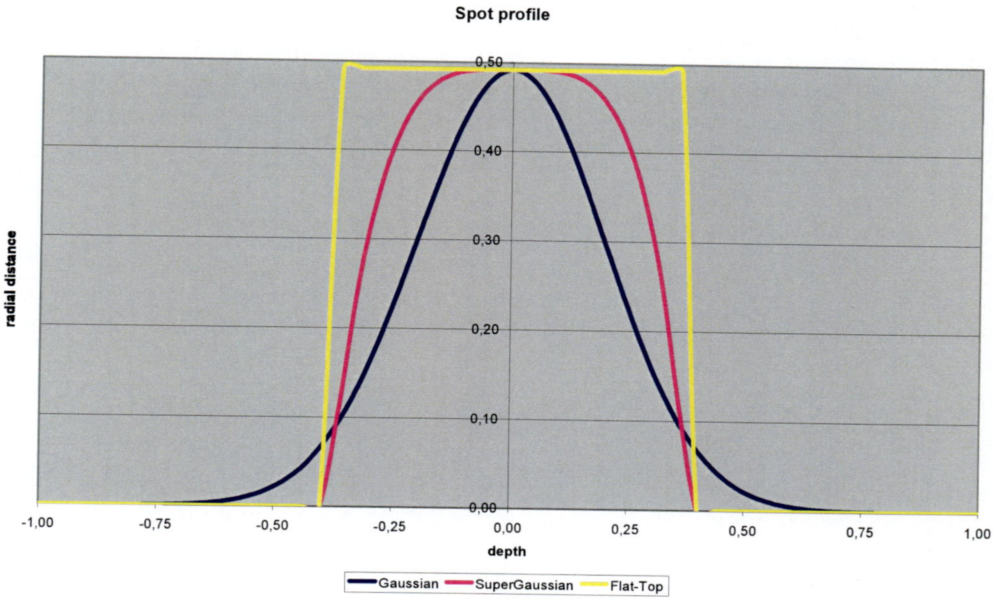


Figure 12. New laser Spot profile modulation (ablation depth distribution): SuperGaussian spot profile corresponding to SCHWIND AMARIS system (in magenta), Flat-Top (Top-Hat) spot profile (in yellow), pure Gaussian spot profile (in blue).

Generating the sequence of laser shot coordinates in a way that:

- guarantees a high fidelity reproduction of the ablation volume line shape
- avoids vacancies and roughness of the cornea
- reduces as much as possible the thermal impact of the ablation by arranging laser shot energy in spatial and temporal distribution
- controls pulse recreation time vs. interspot distance to minimise the heat propagation during the ablation procedure by dynamically limiting the allowed local frequency

Being able to help patients with significant visual problems produces always a great satisfaction, but it is at the same time a major responsibility to treat them with the due respect and very much of care. Nowadays, patients are demanding new and more sophisticated therapeutic strategies, particularly in Laser corneal refractive surgery, to maximise their visual performance.

In this section, we will present strategies concerning wavefront-guided treatments, including in the ablation patterns asymmetric characteristics specific for each individual eye making the ablation more detailed beyond the sphero-cylindrical components.

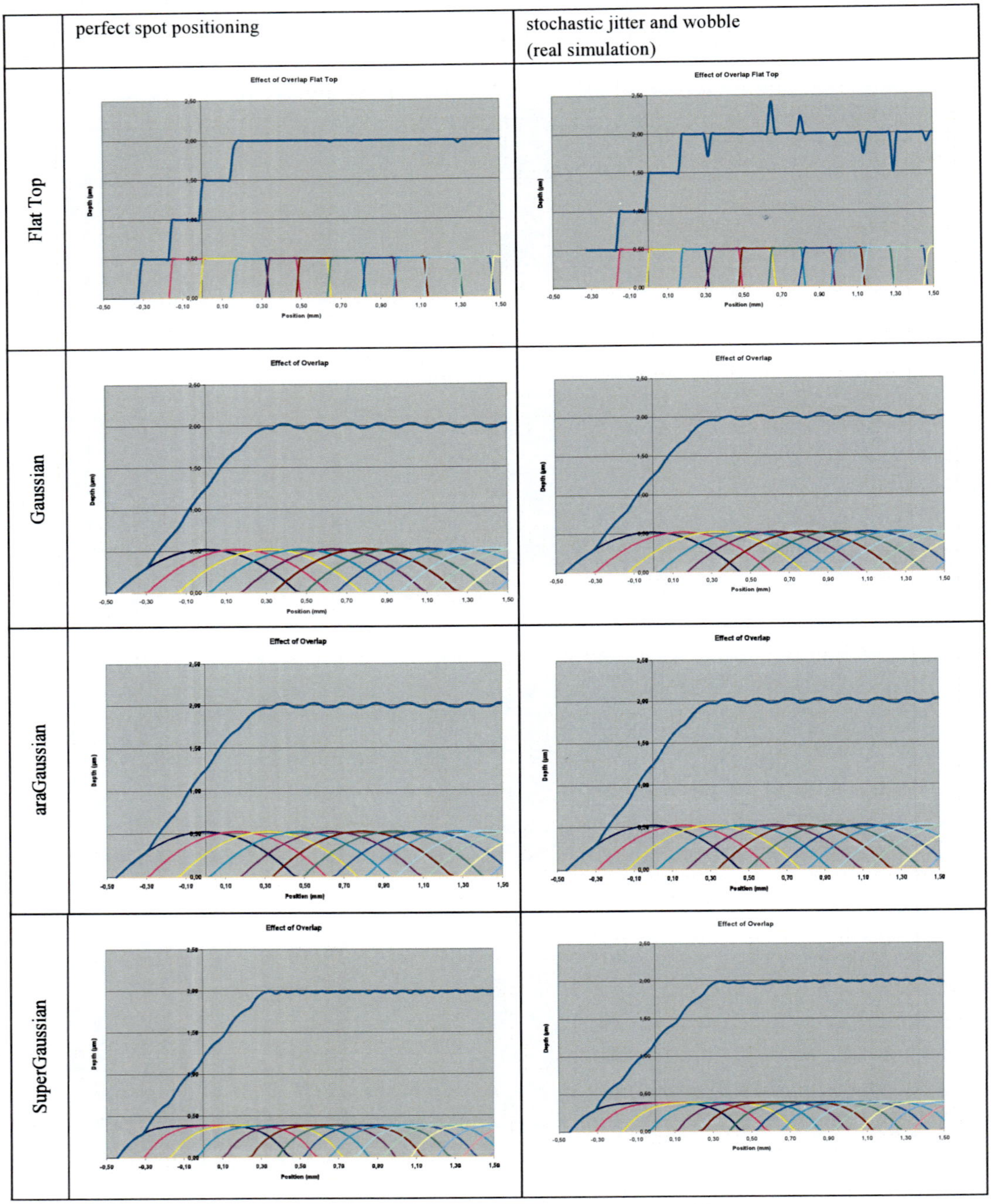


Figure 13. Improved spot overlap matrix guarantees a high fidelity reproduction of the given ablation volume line shape avoiding vacancies and roughness of the cornea. Notice the fidelity differences using Flat-Top (Top-Hat) spot profile (top), pure Gaussian spot profile (middle), paraGaussian spot profile corresponding to ESIRIS system, and superGaussian spot profile corresponding to AMARIS (bottom). Notice as well the stability of paraGaussian and superGaussian spot profiles corresponding to ESIRIS / AMARIS systems by comparing left images (perfect spot positioning) with right images (realistic simulation including stochastic jitter and wobble), compared to the negative overlap effects on Flat-Top (Top-Hat) spot profile (top), and pure Gaussian spot profile (middle).

We will cover ablation profiles guided by topographic information (corneal wavefront treatments) and guided by aberrometric information of the whole eye (ocular wavefront treatments), planning always the most optimum ablation pattern specifically for each individual eye based on its anamnesis, diagnosis, and visual demands.

The optical quality of an eye is significantly determined through its wavefront aberration. This always defines an optical error, regardless of whether it is corneal or ocular wavefront aberration.

SCHWIND eye-tech-solutions has developed its „Wavefront-Guided" treatments for patients whose diagnostically assessed high-order aberrations impair their visual performance, by including corneal and/or ocular wavefront data, allowing a highly individualised, patient-oriented treatment.

With both of the treatment methods, the „Corneal Wavefront guided" as well as the „Ocular Wavefront guided" treatments, the aspherical ablation profile is employed as baseline. These base-lined aspherical ablation profiles of the SCHWIND Custom Ablation Manager (CAM software) compensated induced aberrations through biomechanical influences. Such influences include the microkeratome cut, tissue removal and thinning of the cornea, as well as varying energy losses depending on the corneal curvature during laser correction. These features were already discussed in a previous section.

## Wavefront Guided Treatments with an Aspheric Profile (Schwind CAM - AMARIS / ESIRIS Platform)

Refractive surgery is a rapidly developing industry, which demands technological innovation strength, long-standing application experience and close, continuous co-operation between ophthalmologists and manufacturers. The CAM software is a module developed to import, visualise, and analyse diagnostic data of the eye (manifest refraction, corneal wavefront or ocular wavefront data). Together with additional parameters, to enter manually, an individual ablation volume will be exported to the excimer laser system for the correction of refractive errors.

Based on diagnostic data the CAM software, following advanced algorithms, is capable to integrate ocular wavefront data or topography based corneal wavefront data into the refractive treatment procedure in order to achieve optimum refractive outcomes and visual qualities.

The user interface allows the surgeon to optimize the solution for the patient's problem. The software runs on an independent computer, allowing the surgeon to plan the surgeries in advance without interacting with the excimer laser system.

Figure 14 depicts the increased biomechanical change due to the depth of ablation and due to the corneal layer where they will be ablated. The data showed that it makes not only a difference if the correction is applied to the surface or to the stroma, furthermore the biomechanical response depends on the stromal layer (deeper or more closer to the surface) and their consistence.

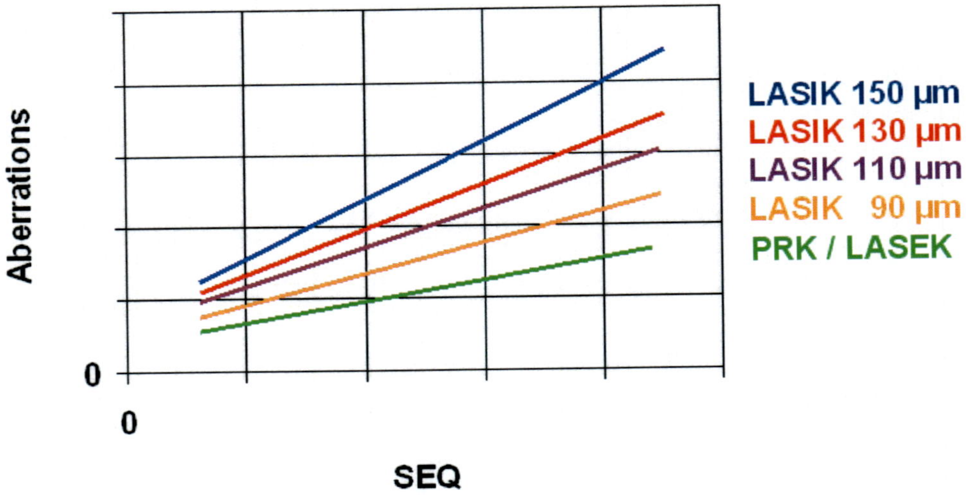


Figure 14. Biomechanical changes due to the ablation, depending on the stromal layer where the tissue will be removed.

## The SCHWIND CAM Software Platform

The ORK-CAM software provides different levels of detail:

- *Aberration-Free treatments:* Based on aspherical profiles, where only the spherical and cylindrical intended refractive change is needed together with the corneal keratometries.

They have the advantage of saving tissue, time and due to their relative simplicity offer a very high predictability

- *Corneal Wavefront treatments*: Based on Corneal Ray Tracing linked to the SCHWIND Corneal Wavefront Analyzer (OPTIKON 2000 spa - Keratron Scout).

They have the advantage of being independent from accommodation effects or light/pupil conditions

- *Ocular Wavefront treatments*: Based on Hartmann-Shack Sensing linked to the SCHWIND Ocular Wavefront Analyzer[67].

They have the advantage of being based on objective refraction of the complete optical system of the human eye

## Key Factors in the CAM Profiles for Customised Treatments:

- Automatic Manifest Refraction Balance

Expected optical impact of the high order aberrations in the refraction is calculated and balanced from the input manifest refraction.

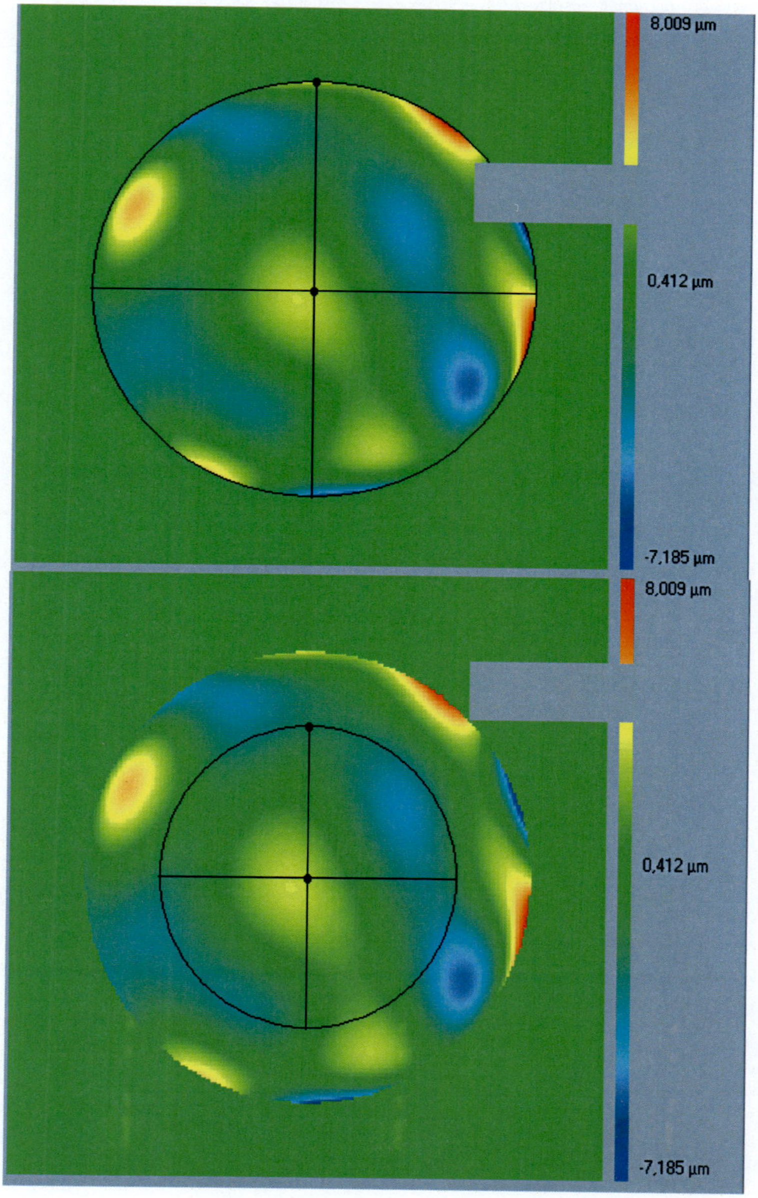

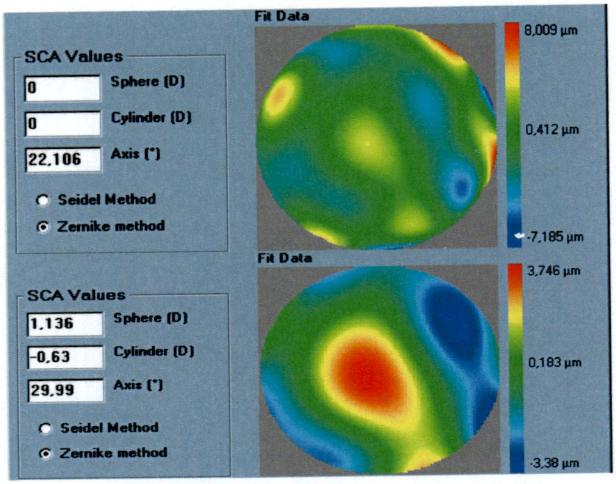


Figure 15. Revolutionary Automatic Manifest Refraction Balance. Expected optical impact of the high order aberrations in the refraction is calculated and balanced from the input manifest refraction. Notice that the same wavefront aberration is analysed for two different diameters. The difference in the refraction provided at the two different analysis diameters correspond to the manifest refraction provided by the high order aberration.

# Optimized Aberration Modes Selection

Based on the wavefront aberration map, the software is able to recommend the best possible aberration modes selection to minimise tissue and time, without compromising the visual quality.

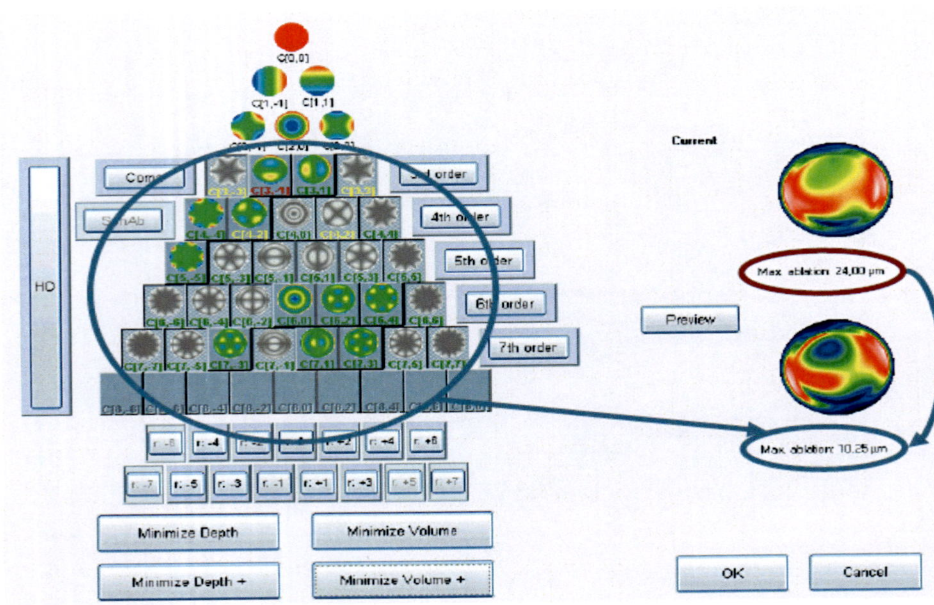

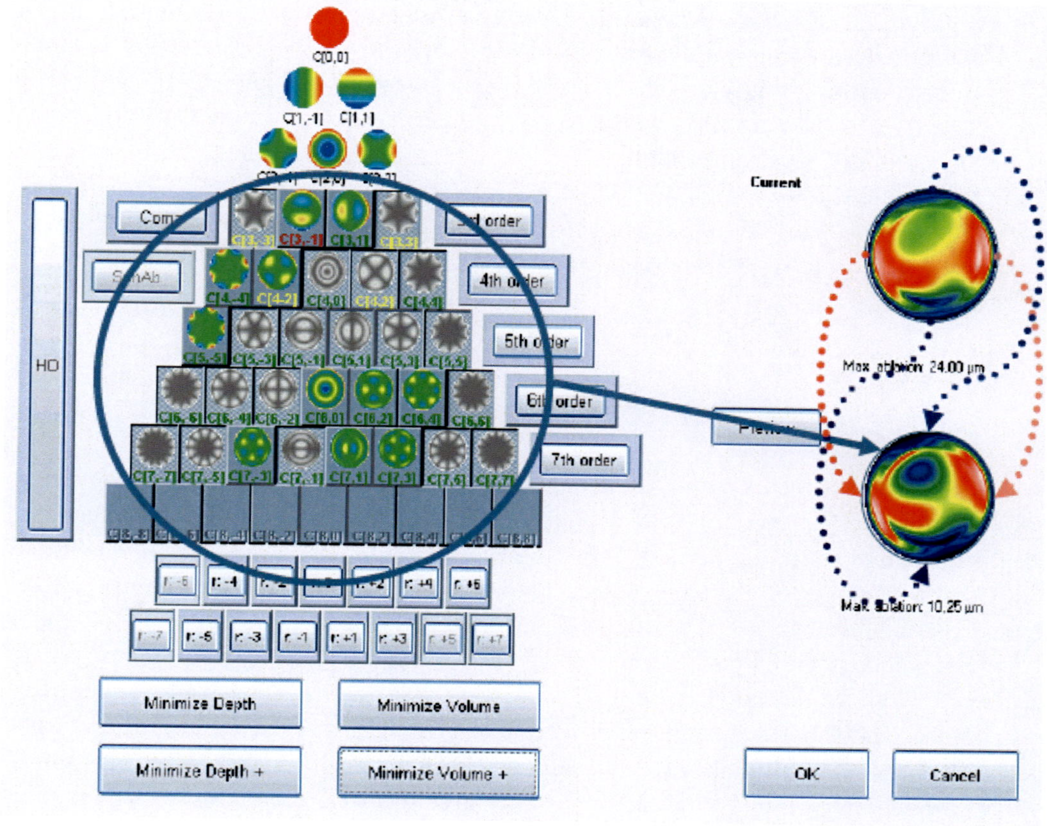


Figure 16. Optimized Aberration Modes Selection. Based on the wavefront aberration map, the software is able to recommend the best possible aberration modes selection to minimise tissue and time, without compromising the visual quality. Notice that the wavefront aberration is analysed by the software showing the original ablation for a full wavefront correction and the suggested set of aberration modes to be corrected. Notice the difference in required tissue, but notice as well that the most representative characteristics of the wavefront map are still presented in the minimised tissue selection.

## Asphericity, Spherical Aberration and the Intended Laser Correction

There is still controversy about the proper definition of an optimal ablation profile for corneal refractive surgery. It has been known for many years that corneal refractive treatments induce a change in corneal asphericity[68] and recently it has been assumed and argued that corneal refractive treatments preserving the preoperative corneal asphericity might be desirable, thus, the asphericity-based profiles have been developed. Topographic-guided, Wavefront-driven, Asphericity preserving and Q-factor profiles have been proposed as ultimate solutions. Nevertheless, considerations as treatment duration, tissue removal, and overall postoperative outcomes make more difficult to establish a universal optimal profile.

- *Corneal Wavefront treatments*: Considering a balanced-eye model (Q-value –0.25) the departure of the measured corneal topography from the theoretically optimal corneal surface was calculated. Optical errors centred on the line-of-sight were described by the Zernike polynomials[69] and the coefficients of the Optical Society of America (OSA) standard[70]
- *Ocular Wavefront treatments*: The high-resolution Hartmann-Shack measurements (~800 points for a 7.2-mm pupil) referred to the entire eye. Optical errors centred on the line-of-sight were described by the Zernike polynomials[69] and the coefficients of the OSA standard[70]

## Corneal Wavefront

The problem of corneal customisation comes from the fact that the real cornea is neither an asphero-toric surface nor a single thin lens system. Topographic systems measure the corneal surface and analyse it through Corneal Ray Tracing to obtain the corneal wavefront error. This wavefront error can be expressed for a given region as a combination of Zernike Polynomials weighted by a set of coefficients, so-called optical aberrations.

Topographic systems use as corneal model a "free-of-spherical-aberration" cornea, which is generated by an aspherical Q-value of $-1/n^2 \sim -0.5$. Nevertheless, statistical analysis over human corneas population has shown as averaged best fitting aspherical surface the one with Q-value around -0.25. Resulting that, in general, the healthy human corneas show a "positive spherical aberration" which is balanced by the "negative spherical aberration" of the internal lens. This aspherical surface with Q-Val -0.25, is the Eye-Model used in the SCHWIND eye-tech-solutions Corneal Wavefront approach.

Comparing the theoretical difference in terms of spherical aberration by using one or another model (Q value $-1/n^2$, Q value -0.25), it is easy to see that the difference depends on both Optical Zone size and K reading. The huger the OZ the bigger the deviation, and the steeper the K reading the bigger the deviation.

Corneal Wavefront is an Advanced Customisation in several senses: combines advantages of Corneal Morphology Customisation, without removing so much tissue (only morphological changes representing optical errors are considered in the approach, thus saving tissue), does not depend primarily on pupil size (topographic coverage use to be huger than pupil size, so we can analyse effects outside actual pupil), is a "stable receptor" (corneal shape does not change so much with age as crystalline lens does).

This Corneal Wavefront profile definition is different from a topography guided profile designed to smooth out corneal surface, where the goal is described with help of a best-fit sphere and in terms of elevation and shape parameters, rather than in terms of wavefront aberration.

Using different input data sources from different devices in refractive surgery most likely lead to some confusion due to the lack of Standards, different Eye Models[71] and different refractive indexes.

We found in the literature different eye models, among others: Eye Models with aspherical Q-Value $-1/n^2$, where n is the refractive index of the cornea, Eye Models with aspherical Q-Value $-1/2n^2$, Eye Models with aspherical Q-Value -0,25. We found also different refractive indices used for the Eye Models, in some cases the keratometric refractive index is used (1,3375), in others different the corneal refractive indices (1,3775 or 1,377 or 1,376 or 1,372), or even sometimes the tear film refractive index (1,336) and a wide range of choices in combination.

Topographic systems measure and analyse the corneal surface as a single thin lens system mostly using keratometric refractive index of 1,3375. Most of the topographic systems use as reference surface an ideal "free-of-aberrations" lens, which is generated by the corresponding Cartesian-Oval[72] (an aspherical surface with Q-Val of $-1/n^2$).

Statistical analysis over human corneas population has shown as average that the best fit aspherical surface the one with Q-Value around -0,25[73,74]. Resulting that in general the healthy human corneas show a "positive spherical aberration" which is balanced by the "negative spherical aberration" of the internal lens. As individuals are aging, the asphericity of the crystalline lens changes, reducing the amount of Spherical aberration that can be balanced or even showing a certain amount of positive spherical aberration, whereas the corneal asphericity thus, corneal spherical aberration, is relatively stable over the time, disrupting the equilibrium between both.

The differences from a Balanced-Eye Model to a Cartesian-Oval Model depend on both Optical Zone size and K-reading. The huger the OZ the bigger is the difference, and the steeper the K-reading the bigger is the difference. As average, one can say that naturally, the human corneas manifest a corneal spherical aberration around 0,23 μm (OSA standard[lxx]).

The first that we should clarify is that these corneal spherical aberrations are not "absolute values" but only in the Topographic system display made under ideal corneal single thin lens approach, referred to a given Cartesian-Oval Model, but they will be different after measurements of the ocular aberrations[75], and definitively close to zero when referred to a Balanced-Eye Model. One can say that the corneal wavefront values in the Topographic system are "overestimated" compared to the ocular wavefront ones.

It is possible to directly calculate the corneal wavefront aberration from the measured surface data. In the case of a rotationally symmetric cornea, the surface shape that will be free of aberrations is a conic surface (aspherical surface) with Q-Val equal to $-1/n^2$ (Cartesian-Oval Model). Any departure from this surface will result in aberrations. The relative elevation of the cornea compared to the best fit Cartesian-Oval Model is the "surface aberration", and if this is known, the corneal wavefront aberration can be computed considering the refractive indices (from Salmon's Dissertation).

However, using a more pragmatic definition, as the corneal surface shape that best represents the averaged human cornea is a conic surface (aspherical surface) with Q-Val equal to -0,25 (Balanced-Eye Model), any departure from this surface can be considered as aberration. The relative elevation of the cornea compared to this Balanced-Eye Model can be considered as the "surface aberration", and the corneal wavefront aberration can be computed.

A Balanced-Eye Model Corneal Wavefront approach is still based on the critical assumption that an aspherical resulting cornea of Q-Value -0,25 will balance its "positive" spherical aberration with the "negative" contribution of the internal lens (which is true only in average for the non-treated population[73,74,76]). Opposite, one can also propose, as alternative, using as reference corneal surface the best fit aspherical Q-Value for each individual cornea. This will lead also to the critical assumption that the overall "Ocular" spherical aberration for each individual eye is close-to-zero (which is also true only in average for the non-treated population[77]).

Corneal spherical aberration directly depends upon the selected model eye used for the simulated ray tracing.

## Ocular Wavefront Treatments

The diagnosis should always be as detailed as possible, "combining" the information coming from Topographic systems (K-reading, Asphericity, Corneal Wavefront Aberration) with the information coming from Aberrometer systems (Objective refraction, Ocular Wavefront Aberration) will give us better possibility to decide which kind of treatment we choose. Anyway, special care should be taken with expressions such as "induced wavefront components less than 0,25 μm are not clinically relevant", where basic information is missing (of course Standard used and Optical Zone size, but also data source and Eye Model, if used).

The standard parameters used to assess refractive surgery results (efficacy, predictability, refractive outcome, stability, and safety) are not sufficient to evaluate the optimal customisation approach.

When comparing and evaluating the outcomes of two different wavefront customisation strategies, wavefront aberration analysis is mandatory to determine whether the customisation aims have been achieved.

Wavefront customised treatments (either Corneal Wavefront or Ocular Wavefront) can only be successful if the pre-existing aberrations are greater than the repeatability, biological noise, and accommodation effects. Considerations such as treatment duration or tissue removal make it more difficult to establish a universal optimal profile as follows:

- *Aberration-Free* treatments have the advantage of saving tissue and time, and due to their simplicity, they offer better predictability
- *Corneal Wavefront* treatments have the advantage of being independent from accommodation effects or light/pupil conditions
- *Ocular Wavefront* treatments have the advantage of being based on objective refraction of the complete human eye system

The SCHWIND CAM wavefront-guided profiles were developed with the aim of producing "aberration-free" optics, compensating the preoperative existing wavefront aberration (within the OZ).

Wavefront-guided treatments are not always the "gold standard". Moreover, optimal refractive surgery is generally achieved by balancing the effects on wavefront aberration and providing normal eyes with the best quality of vision without affecting their perception of the world.

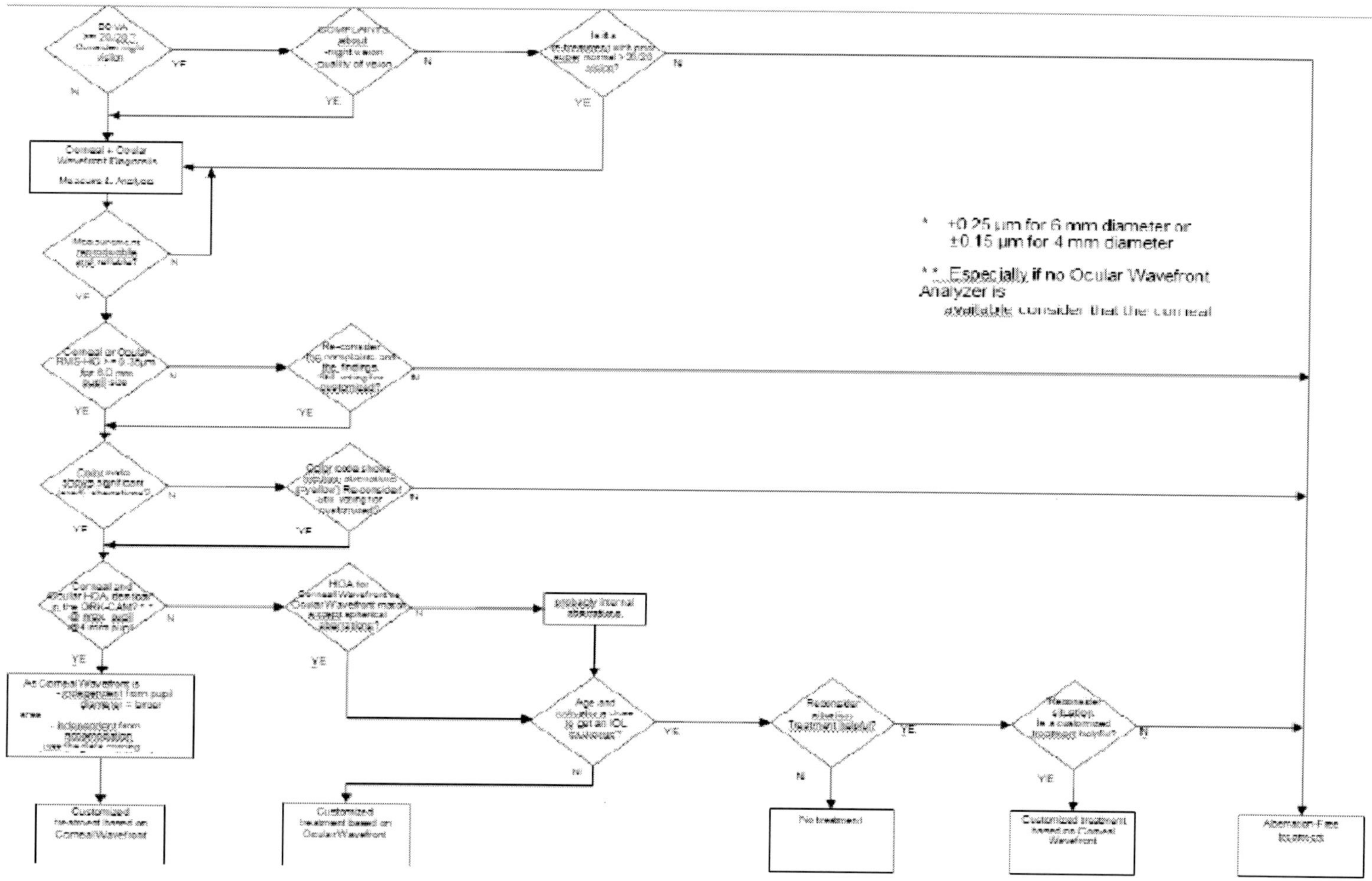


Figure 17. Decision-tree to find the kind of corneal refractive surgery from which the individual patient will benefit most.

Aspheric Corneal Wavefront treatments or Ocular Wavefront treatments ablation profiles, designed with CAM software for the AMARIS / ESIRIS laser platform, yielded visual, optical, and refractive results comparable to those of other wavefront-guided customised techniques. No significant differences in the comparative outcomes of both customised strategies exist. Moreover, an absolute optimal strategy has not been found, and "aberration-free" optimized ablation generally represents a less time-consuming approach than the wavefront customised approaches, as it is based on preoperative manifest refraction, which is mandatory for detecting refractive disorders. The "aberration-free" optimized profile therefore has the potential to replace currently used standard profiles for refractive corrections. The CW and OW customised approaches show their strengths in cases where abnormal optical systems are expected. It is clear that treating all patients systematically with wavefront-customised approaches carries no risk other than the extra tissue requirement for ablation. Thus, as a general classification, we would propose the following:

- *Aberration-free* treatments for eyes with a BSCVA ≥20/20 and no symptomatic aberrations that require primary corneal laser refractive treatments
- *Corneal Wavefront* treatments for eyes with symptomatic aberrations with a BSCVA <20/20 that require corneal laser refractive re-treatments
- *Ocular Wavefront* treatments for eyes with a BSCVA <20/20 or symptomatic aberrations that require primary corneal laser refractive treatments

Nevertheless to come closer to an answer about the questions "From which kind of corneal refractive laser surgery will my patient benefit most?" a flow chart as proposed in Figure 17 might be a very helpful tool.

As we noticed, there is more than one criterion, which votes for Aberration-Free or for Corneal / Ocular Wavefront guided. Besides of this proposed flow chart other circumstances should be considered like the risks arising from the different methods of treatments, your diagnostic findings and at least do not forget your personal experience.

# References

[1] Levy Y, Segal O, Avni I, Zadok D. Ocular higher-order aberrations in eyes with supernormal vision. *American Journal of Ophthalmology*; 2005; 139: 225-228

[2] Artal P. What aberration pattern (if any) produces the best vision?, 6th International Wavefront Congress, Athens, Greece; February 2005

[3] Artal P, Chen L, Fernández EJ, Singer B, Manzanera S, Williams DR. Neural compensation for the eye's optical aberrations. *Journal of Vision*; 2004; 4:281-287

[4] Held R. The rediscovery of adaptability in the visual system: effects of extrinsic and intrinsic chromatic dispersion. In Harris CS, ed. Visual coding and Adaptability. Hillsdalle, NJ: Lawrence Erbaum Associates; 1980

[5] Awwad ST, El-Kateb M, Bowman RW et al. Wavefront-guided Laser in situ keratomileusis with the Alcon CustomCornea and the VISX CustomVue: Three month results. *J Refract Surg* 2004; 20:S636-S643

[6] Buhren J, Kohnen T. Factors affecting the change in lower-order and higher-order aberrations after wavefront-guided laser in situ keratomileusis for myopia with the Zyoptix 3.1 system. *J Cataract Refract Surg*; 2006; 32: 1166-74

[7] Munnerlyn CR, Koons SJ, Marshall J. Photorefractive keratectomy: a technique for laser refractive surgery. *J Cataract Refract Surg*; 1988;14:46–52

[8] Mrochen M, Kaemmerer M, Seiler T. Clinical results of wavefront-guided laser in situ keratomileusis 3 months after surgery. *J Cataract Refract Surg*. 2001;27:201-7.

[9] Mattioli R, Tripoli NK. Corneal Geometry Reconstruction with the Keratron Videokeratographer. *Optometry and Vision Science* 1997; 74: 881-94

[10] Salmon TO. Corneal contribution to the Wavefront aberration of the eye. *PhD Dissertation*; 1999:70

[11] Salmon T. Measurement of Refractive Errors in Young Myopes using the COAS Shack-Hartmann Aberrometer. *Optometry and Vision Science;*2003;Vol 80

[12] Trokel SL, Srinivasan R, Braren B. Excimer laser surgery of the cornea. *Am J Ophthalmol*. 1983; 96:710-5

[13] Marshall J, Trokel S, Rothery S, Schubert H. An ultrastructural study of corneal incisions induced by an excimer laser at 193 nm. Ophthalmology. 1985; 92:749-58

[14] Marcos S, Cano D, Barbero S. Increase in corneal asphericity after standard laser in situ keratomileusis for myopia is not inherent to the Munnerlyn algorithm. *J Refract Surg*; 2003;19:S592-6

[15] Moreno-Barriuso E, Lloves JM, Marcos S. Ocular Aberrations before and after myopic corneal refractive surgery: LASIK-induced changes measured with LASER ray tracing. *Invest Ophthalmol Vis Sci* 2001; 42:1396-1403

[16] Anera RG, Jiménez JR, Jiménez del Barco L, Bermúdez J, Hita E. Changes in corneal asphericity after refractive surgery. *Journal of Cataract and Refractive Surgery* 2003; 29: 762-768

[17] Yoon G, MacRae S, Williams DR, Cox IG. Causes of spherical aberration induced by laser refractive surgery. *J Cataract Refract Surg;* 2005;31:127-135

[18] Mrochen M, Seiler T. Influence of Corneal Curvature on Calculation of Ablation Patterns used in photorefractive Laser Surgery. *J Refract Surg;* 2001;17:584-587

[19] Jiménez JR, Anera RG, Jiménez del Barco L, Hita E. Effect on laser-ablation algorithms of reflection losses and nonnormal incidence on the anterior cornea. *Applied Physics Letters;* 2002;81;8:1521-1523

[20] Jiménez JR, Anera RG, Jiménez del Barco L, Hita E, Pérez-Ocón F. Correlation factor for ablation agorithms used in corneal refractive surgery with gaussian-profile beams. *Optics Express;* 2005;13;1:336-343

[21] Dorronsoro C, Cano D, Merayo-Lloves J, Marcos S. Experiments on PMMA models to predict the impact of corneal refractive surgery on corneal shape. *Optics Express;* 2006; 14: 6142-6156

[22] Roberts C. The cornea is not a piece of plastic. *J Refract Surg*; 2000; 16: 407-13

[23] Thibos L, Bradley A, Applegate R. Accuracy and precision of objective refraction from wavefront aberrations. *ISSN 1534-7362* , 2003 ARVO

[24] Liang J, Grimm B, Goelz S, Bille JF. Objective measurement of wave aberrations of the human eye with the use of a Hartmann-Shack wave-front sensor. J Opt Soc Am A Opt Image Sci Vis. 1994;11: 1949-57

[25] Alio JL, Belda JI, Osman AA, Shalaby AM. Topography-guided laser in situ keratomileusis (TOPOLINK) to correct irregular astigmatism after previous refractive surgery. *J Refract Surg*; 2003;19:516-27.

[26] Mrochen M, Jankov M, Bueeler M, Seiler T. Correlation Between Corneal and Total Wavefront Aberrations in Myopic Eyes. *J Refract Surg;* 2003;19:104-112

[27] Arbelaez MC. Super vision: dream or reality. *J Refract Surg*. 2001;17: S211-8

[28] Wigledowska-Promienska D, Zawojska I. Changes in higher order aberrations after wavefront-guided PRK for correction of low to moderate myopia and myopic astigmatism: two-year follow-up. *Eur J Ophthalmol*. 2007; 17:507-14

[29] Huang D, Arif M. Spot size and quality of scanning laser correction of higher-order wavefront aberrations. *J Cataract Refract Surg;* 2002;28:407-416

[30] Guirao A,Williams D, MacRae S. Effect of beam size on the Expected benefit of customized laser refractive surgery. *J Refract Surg;* 2003;19:15-23

[31] Taylor NM, Eikelboom RH, van Sarloos PP, Reid PG. Determining the accuracy of an eye tracking system for laser refractive surgery. *J Refract Surg*. 2000; 16: S643-6

[32] Bueeler M, Mrochen M. Simulation of eye-tracker latency, spot size, and ablation pulse depth on the correction of higher order wavefront aberrations with scanning spot laser systems. *J Refract Surg*; 2005; 21: 28-36

[33] Smith EM Jr, Talamo JH. Cyclotorsion in the seated and the supine patient. *J Cataract Refract Surg* 1995; 21:402-403.

[34] Porter J, Yoon G, MacRae S, Pan G, Twietmeyer T, Cox IG, Williams DR. Surgeon offsets and dynamic eye movements in laser refractive surgery. *J Cataract Refract Surg*. 2005; 31: 2058-66

[35] Guirao A, Williams D, Cox I. Effect of rotation and translation on the expected benefit of an ideal method to correct the eyes higher-order aberrations. *J.Opt.Soc.Am.A;*2001;18:1003-1015

[36] Bueeler M, Mrochen M. Limitations of pupil tracking in refractive surgery: systematic error in determination of corneal locations. *J Refract Surg*. 2004;20: 371-8

[37] Avetisov SE, Karamian AA, Sukhanova EV. [Indications for optimized refractive keratoablation. Communication 1. Dependence on the grade of myopia and baseline high-order aberrations] *Vestn Oftalmol*. 2007;123: 3-5

[38] Avetisov SE, Karamian AA, Sukhanova EV. [Indications for optimized refractive keratoablation. Communication 2. Dependence on baseline spherical aberrations] *Vestn Oftalmol*. 2007; 123: 6-8

[39] Karamian AA, Sukhanova EV. [Evaluation of the efficiency of aspheric eximer laser keratoablation (a preliminary communication)] *Vestn Oftalmol*. 2007; 123: 20-2

[40] Karamian AA, Sukhanova EV. [Comparative clinical study of the standard lasik operation versus optimized ORK "Corwave" keratoablation (a preliminary communication)] *Vestn Oftalmol*. 2006; 122:6-8

[41] Calossi A. Corneal asphericity and spherical aberration. *J Refract Surg*. 2007; 23: 505-14

[42] Lipshitz I. Thirty-four Challenges to Meet Before Excimer Laser Technology Can Achieve Super Vision. *J Refract Surg;* 2002;18:740-743

[43] Tran DB, Sarayba MA, Bor Z, Garufis C, Duh YJ, Soltes CR, Juhasz T, Kurtz RM. Randomized prospective clinical study comparing induced aberrations with IntraLase and Hansatome flap creation in fellow eyes. *J Cataract Refract Surg;* 2005;31:97-105

[44] Durrie DS, Kezirian GM. Femtosecond laser versus mechanical keratome flaps in wavefront-guided laser in situ keratomileusis. *J Cataract Refract Surg;* 2005;31:120-126

[45] Huang D, Arif M. Spot size and quality of scanning laser correction of higher-order wavefront aberrations. *J Cataract Refract Surg;* 2002;28:407-416

[46] Guirao A,Williams D, MacRae S. Effect of beam size on the Expected benefit of customized laser refractive surgery. *J Refract Surg;* 2003;19:15-23

[47] Bueeler M, Mrochen M. Simulation of Eye-tracker Latency, Spot Size, and Ablation Pulse Depth on the Correction of Higher Order Wavefront Aberrations With Scanning Spot Laser Systems. *J Refract Surg;* 2005;21:28-36

[48] Schruender S, Fuchs H, Spasovski S, Dankert A. Intraoperative Corneal Topography for Image Registration. *J Refract Surg;* 2002;18:S624-S629

[49] Bueeler M, Mrochen M. Limitations of Pupil Tracking in Refractive Surgery: systematic Error in Determination of Corneal Locations. *J Refract Surg;* 2004;20:371-378

[50] Roberts C, Dupps WJ. Corneal biomechanics and their role in corneal ablative procedures. McRae SM Krueger RR Applegate RA eds. *Customized Corneal Ablation: The Quest for Supervision. Wavefront Standards.* 2000;109-131. Slack Inc Thorofare, NJ

[51] Marcos S, Cano D, Barbero S. Increase in corneal asphericity after standard laser in situ keratomileusis for myopia is not inherent to the Munnerlyn algorithm. *J Refract Surg*; 2003;19:S592-6

[52] Mastropasqua L, Toto L, Zuppardi E, Nubile M, Carpineto P, Di Nicola M, Ballone E. Photorefractive keratectomy with aspheric profile of ablation versus conventional photorefractive keratectomy for myopia correction: six-month controlled clinical trial. *J Cataract Refract Surg*; 2006;32:109-16

[53] Koller T, Iseli HP, Hafezi F, Mrochen M, Seiler T. Q-factor customized ablation profile for the correction of myopic astigmatism. *J Cataract Refract Surg;* 2006; 32:584-589

[54] De Ortueta, Arba-Mosquera S. Mathematical properties of Asphericity: A Method to calculate with asphericities. *Journal of Refractive Surgery. (In press)*

[55] Antonio Calossi. The optical quality of the cornea. Fabiano Editore 2002

[56] Patel S, Marshall J, Fitzke FW. Model for predicting the optical performance of the eye in refractive surgery. *Refract Corneal Surg*; 1993;9:366-75.

[57] Manns F, Ho H, Parel JM, Culbertson W. Ablation profiles for wavefront-guided correction of myopia and primary spherical aberration. *J Cataract Refract Surg*; 2002;28:766–774

[58] Díaz JA, Anera RG, Jiménez JR, Jiménez del Barco L. Optimum corneal asphericity of myopic eyes for refractive surgery, *Journal of Modern Optics;* 2003; 50:1903-1915

[59] Somani S, Tuan KA, Chernyak D. Proceedings of the 5th International Congress of Wavefront Sensing and Optimized Refractive Corrections: Corneal Asphericity and Retinal Image Quality: A Case Study and Simulations. *J Refract Surg* 2004; 20: S581-S585

[60] Pallikaris IG, Siganos DS. Excimer laser in situ keratomileusis and photorefractive keratectomy for correction of high myopia. J Refract Corneal Surg. 1994; 10: 498-510

[61] Pettit, G H; Ediger, M N. Corneal-tissue absorption coefficients for 193- and 213-nm ultraviolet radiation. *Applied Optics*, 1996; 35: 3386-3391

[62] Barbero S, Refractive power of a multilayer rotationally symmetric model of the human cornea and tear film. J. Opt. Soc. Am. A 2006; 23: 1578-1585

[63] Gatinel D, Hoang-Xuan T. Geometric customization of optical and transition zone parameters for treatment of compound myopic astigmatism with the NIDEK EC-5000 excimer laser. *J Refract Surg*. 2007; 23: 924-30

[64] Zaldivar R, Oscherow S, Bains HS. Five techniques for improving outcomes of hyperopic LASIK. *J Refract Surg*. 2005; 21: S628-32

[65] Bará S, Mancebo T, Moreno-Barriuso E. Positioning Tolerances for Phase Plates Compensating Aberrations of the Human Eye. *Appl. Opt.* 2000; 39: 3413-3420

[66] Wygledowska-Promieńska D, Zawojska I, Gierek-Ciaciura S. [Evaluation of eye total aberration in patients after PRK and LASIK procedures] Klin Oczna. 2004;106(4-5):637-42

[67] Salmon T. Measurement of Refractive Errors in Young Myopes using the COAS Shack-Hartmann Aberrometer. *Optometry and Vision Science;*2003;Vol 80.

[68] Anera RG, Jiménez JR, Jiménez del Barco L, Bermúdez J, Hita E, Changes in corneal asphericity after LASER in situ keratomileusis, *J Cataract Refract Surg;* 2003; 29:762-768

[69] Zernike F. Diffraction theory of the knife-edge test and its improved form, the phase-contrast method. *Physica I;* 1934;689-704

[70] Thibos LN, Applegate RA, Schwiegerling JT, Webb R, VSIA Standards Taskforce Members. Standards for reporting the optical aberrations of eyes. *J Refract Surg;* 2002;18:S652-S660

[71] Thibos L, Bradley A. Modeling the Refractive and Neuro-Sensor Systems of the Eye. *VISUAL INSTRUMENTATION:Chapter 4;*1999;101-159

[72] Clarkson ENK, Levi-Setti R. Trilobite eyes and the optics of Descartes and Huygens. *Nature* 1975;254:663-7

[73] Kiely PM, Smith G, Carney LG. The mean shape of the human cornea. *Optica Acta.* 1982;29:1027-1040

[74] Sheridan M, Douthwaite WA. Corneal asphericity and refractive error. *Ophthal Physiol Opt* 1989;9:235-238

[75] Marcos S, Barbero S, Llorente L, Merayo-Lloves J. Optical response to LASIK surgery for myopia from Total and Corneal Aberration Measurements. *Invest Ophthalmol Vis Sci;* 2001;42:3349-3356

[76] Antonio Calossi. The optical quality of the cornea. Fabiano Editore 2002

[77] Thibos LN, Hong X, Bradley A, Cheng X. Statistical variation of aberration structure and image quality in a normal population of healthy eyes. *J Opt Soc Am A Opt Image Sci Vis;* 2002;19:2329-48.

In: Laser Keratectomy: Approaches, Complications... ISBN 978-1-60456-863-9
Author: Luis W. Schröder and Felix J. Walter 

*Chapter VII*

# Amblyopia and Refractive Surgery

***A. Fea, F. Tofani, A. Morra, G. Strani, and F.M. Grignolo***
Dipartimento di Fisiopatologia Clinica, Clinica Oculistica,
Universita' di Torino-Italy

Amblyopia is one of the most common preventable causes of visual acuity loss in children.The Amblyopia Treatment Studies[1] (ATS) report excellent results in reversing amblyopia with glasses in combination with patching, atropine treatment, or both. Conversely, the ATS studies also show that a significant subset of amblyopic patients, even without coexisting medical or ocular problems, do not have successful, timely resolution of their amblyopia with standard treatment regimens. Recently refractive surgery has been proposed in addition to standard antiamblyopic treatments, especially in patients with high refractive errors and non compliant with contact lens use.

## Adults

Surgical treatment of amblyogenic refractive errors in adults who should have already completed the development of vision is controversial. The existing reports regarding laser refractive surgery in amblyopic eyes refer mainly to the pediatric population and include only a small number of eyes. Informations on adult patients are limited to 4 studies (2 LASIK ; 2 PRK).

Recently, Barequet et al [2] reported encouraging visual and refractive results in adult patients with amblyopia treated with LASIK . Eight eyes were included, with a mean patient age of 30 +/- 10 years (range 21 to 49 yr). Mean preoperative spherical equivalent refraction was -4.70 D (range -12.62 to +4.71 D) and the best spectacle-corrected visual acuity varied from 20/32 to 20/80. At 2 months after LASIK, mean spherical equivalent refraction was -0.37 +/- 0.60 D (range -1.37 to + 0.60 D), uncorrected visual acuity ranged between 20/20 to 20/30, and a mean gain of 3 Snellen lines (range 2 to 4 lines) was observed. From 2 to 6 months mean spheric equivalent (SE) ranged between -1.00 to +1.00 D with an astigmatism range between -0.25 and -1.25 D. The visual acuity and subjective improvement were maintained throughout the 6 month postoperative period. All patients reported significant subjective improvement.

In a retrospective study Sakatani et al [3] considered 21 eyes of 19 patients (22-26 yrs; 7F, 12M) identified as having amblyopia and LASIK surgery. Eight patients (42.1%) were diagnosed with amblyopia only, 6 patients (31.6%) had anisometropic amblyopia, 4 patients (21.1%) had strabismic amblyopia, and 1 patient (5.2%) had anisometropic and strabismic amblyopia. Two patients had bilateral amblyopia.

Eleven eyes (52.4%) had myopic astigmatism, 7 eyes (33.3%) were hyperopic, and 3 eyes (14.3%) had mixed astigmatism. Mean spherical equivalent ranged between -3.00 and +6.75 D with astigmatism between +0.50 and +3.75 D. mean preoperative BSCVA was 20/35 (range 20/300 to 20/20 ). The mean postoperative UCVA was 20/33 (range 20/200 to 20/20) and the mean postoperative BSCVA, 20/29 (range 20/200 to 20/15). Seven eyes (33.3 %) experienced more than a 1-line improvement in postoperative UCVA compared with the preoperative BSCVA. Nine eyes (42.8%) experienced more than a 1-line improvement in postoperative BSCVA compared with the preoperative BSCVA. The BSCVA was unchanged in 11 eyes (52.4%) and was worse by 2 lines in 1 eye (4.8%). In one eye a second LASIK treatment was done to compensate the loss of 2 lines due to epithelial ingrowth.

Improvement in BSCVA was statistically significant in eyes that had strabismic amblyopia , in patients who received treatment for amblyopia as children, in patients who previously were contact lens wearers and in amblyopic eyes with myopia but not in amblyopic eyes with hyperopia or mixed astigmatism.

In a restrospective study by Lanza et al [4], 38 amblyopic eyes of 36 adult patients were considered. Patients' ages at the time of refractive surgery ranged between 20 and 59 years, spherical equivalent ranged from 14.63 to 3.75 D, astigmatism ranged between -5.00 and +4.50 D. Thirty eyes had compound myopic astigmatism; 1 eye, myopia; 5 eyes, mixed astigmatism; and 2 eyes, hyperopia. Two of the patients had bilateral amblyopia. The causes of amblyopia were strabismic amblyopia in 14 eyes, isometropic amblyopia in 4 eyes, and anisometropic amblyopia in 20 eyes.

Before PRK, BSCVA ranged between 0.2 and 0.7 lines . One month after PRK, BSCVA ranged between 0.2 and 1.2 lines. Three months after PRK, BSCVA ranged between 0.15 and 1.15 lines

Six months after PRK, BSCVA ranged between 0.25 and 1.3 lines. At 6-month follow-up, 17 of 19 examined eyes (89%) gained 1 line, and of these,13 (68%) gained 2 lines.

Best results were obtained after six months, in patients with mild to moderate amblyopia,in younger patients and in the eyes that achieved a better astigmatic correction.

These studies have limitations. First of all they are retrospective, secondly they focus on refraction and often the orthoptic examination and information on previous antiamblyopic treatments is lacking. The majority of treated patients is myopic and it is not possibile to determine if VA increase is due to resolution of amblyopia or to an increase in image size after treatment. Long term follow up is also missing and it is not possibile to determine if results obtained are stable.

Recent studies by El Mallah et al [5] show that functional recovery may be partially due to an increase in cortical recruitment, in fact older people with a history of amblyopia who develop visual loss in the previously normal eye can experience recovery of visual function in the amblyopic eye over a period of time. This recovery in visual function occurs in the event of visual loss in the fellow eye and the improvement appears to be sustained over time.

Recently, Roszkowska et al[6] performed an interventional study on 50 patients with amblyopia treated with photorefractive keratectomy. Sixty-eight eyes of 18 participants with bilateral refractive amblyopia and 32 participants with unilateral anisometropic amblyopia were studied.

In 64.7% of eyes, the UCVA at 12 months after the treatment was better than or equal to their preoperative BCVA. A total of 82.4% of eyes improved their BCVA one or more lines. No eye lost lines of BCVA, 17.6% remained unvaried, 50% gained one line, 20.6

% gained two lines, and 11.8% gained three lines of BCVA. The mean spere changed from –5.62±3.37 D to –0.47±1 D, mean cylinder varied from –2.36±1.57 to –0.18±0.41 D, and the spherical equivalent varied from –6.82±3.1 to –0.45±1.08 D. No clinically significant haze was observed . The most important data obtained in this study are related to the group of patients with anisometropia. In fact a significant correlation between diopters of anisometropia and visual improvement was demonstrated, therefore high dioptric differences led to high visual recovery in eyes with anisometropic amblyopia.

Widespread use of refractive surgery in adult amblyopic patients will need to be further investigated possibly in controlled studies.

## Children

A major contribution to the discussion of parameters for considering a patient to be at significant risk for developing amblyopia was recently published by France[7] . This paper outlines the evidence-based guidelines that are the most helpful in screening for amblyogenic potential. They are hyperopia greater than 3.50 D in any meridian, myopia greater than 3.00 D in any meridian, astigmatism greater than 1.50 D at 90 or 180 degrees, astigmatism greater than 1.00 D in an oblique axis, and anisometropia (spherical or cylindrical) greater than 1.50 D.

Refractive surgery for children with significant refractive errors remains a field of investigation. Surgical intervention is often reserved for children with severe and refractory amblyopia secondary to high anisometropia, high myopia and poor compliance with conventional spectacle and/or contact lens correction and amblyopia therapy. Failure of traditional amblyopia treatments may be especially true in children with coexisting medical diagnoses such as autism, cerebral palsy, developmental delay, and other ocular disorders.[8] In a study by Nucci et al[9] 14 eyes of 14 patients with unilateral high myopia (9-14 years age range) underwent PRK (11 eyes) or LASIK (3 eyes) on the more myopic eye under topical anesthesia. The postoperative regimen for PRK included wearing a soft contact lens for 4 days after the procedure and applying tobramycin twice a day for 5 days. Fluorometholon eye drops were used for up to 4 months, with the dosage titrated to severity of signs and symptoms. Artificial tears were prescribed for use 3 to 4 times a day for 2 months. The regimen for LASIK included applying tobramycin twice a day for 5 days and fluorometholon for up to 3 weeks. Artificial tears were prescribed 3 to 4 times a day for 2 months.

The average age at the time of surgery was 11.9±1,6 years. The average corrected preoperative visual acuity was 0.14±0.065, the average preoperative SE was –7.96±2,16 D . Twenty months after refractive surgery, the uncorrected visual acuity averaged 0.16±0.08 and best corrected vision averaged 0.17±0.08. The average refraction was –0.46±0,58 D at 2 months and –0.67±0,68 D at 20 months (-0.87D with LASIK and -0.02 with PRK). LASIK patients averaged –0.875 D of myopic shift over 20 months of follow-up. Those with PRK averaged –0.025 D. The vision of 5 of 14 patients improved 1 or 2 lines after refractive surgery. Two patients with 20/80 vision preoperatively improved to 20/60. No patients lost lines of vision. Only 4 patients demonstrated stereopsis preoperatively, and all retained stereopsis postoperatively. No patient gained stereopsis. This could be related to the fact that patients had already passed the critical period for stereopsis development. LASIK and PRK can be performed safely and effectively in children who are cooperative enough to undergo the procedures under topical anesthesia. Refractive surgery does not improve vision in densely amblyopic eyes but may give modest improvement in patients with mild amblyopia.

No serious complications occurred, no patient developed a new strabismus or diplopia; no patient with preoperative strabismus became orthophoric.

The refractive status of some pediatric patients with bilateral high myopia and unilateral myopic anisometropic amblyopia is not successfully treated with traditional methods, including glasses and contact lenses. When these children have a concurrent medical diagnosis such as autism, cerebral palsy, and developmental delay associated with other coexisting ocular disorders (including cornea, retina, and optic nerve disorders), visual rehabilitation may be impossible. Patients with significant developmental delay or behavior abnormalities that preclude the use of glasses or contact lenses are also potential candidates for refractive surgery9.

Astle et al[10] performed PRK in 40 eyes of 27 patients 1 to 6 years of age. Thirty three percent of patients had had some comorbidity, such as cerebral palsy, ex-prematurity, autism, and developmental delay The patients were divided into 4 groups based on the type of myopia: myopic anisometropic amblyopia (15 eyes/13 patients), bilateral high myopia (20 eyes/10 patients), high myopia post-penetrating keratoplasty (3 eyes/2 patients), and combined corneal scarring and anisometropic amblyopia (2 eyes/2 patients). All procedures were performed under general anesthesia. The mean SE decreased from 10.68 D to 1.37 D at 1 year, a mean change of 9.31 D. At 1 year, the mean best corrected visual acuity improved from 20/70 to 20/40 in the entire group. Fourty percent of eyes were within 1.0 D of the targeted refraction. There was no haze in 59.5% of eyes. Binocular vision increased in 64% of patients. A functional vision survey demonstrated a positive effect on the children's ability to function in their environments after the laser treatment.

Autrata et al[11] conducted a prospective comparative study on 27 children (mean age 5.4 yrs; range 4 to 7 yrs) intolerant to contact lenses, with high myopic anisometropia and amblyopia. Multizonal PRK (13 eyes) or LASEK (14 eyes) was performed in the more myopic eye under general anesyhesia. As the patients could not fixate on the aiming beam, the center of the pupil was chosen as the most appropriate center for the beam. After surgery, the dominant eye was patched. All children had a 2-year follow-up. The 27 children (group A) were compared with a control group of 30 children (group B, mean age 5.1 years) in whom myopic anisometropia and amblyopia were treated conventionally by CLs and patching of the dominant eye.

In Group A, the mean spherical equivalent refraction was -8.25 ± 2.37 D (range -6.00 to -11.25 D) preoperatively and -1.61 ± 1.13 D (range +0.75 to -2.25 D) postoperatively. A 96% reduction in anisometropia and stable results were observed during follow up. In Group A 25% of patients gained 1 to 3 Snellen lines, 53.4% gained 4 to 8 lines. Twenty-two children were supplemented with spectacles for the residual refractive error. Axial length increased during the follow up in both groups without significant differences. In the control group only 20% gained 4 to 8 lines and 50% 1 to 3 lines.

The mean BCVA was 0.23 ± 0.21 preoperatively and 0.78 ± 0.19 at 2 years. In Group B, the mean BCVA was 0.16 ± 0.19 at the start of CL correction and amblyopia therapy and improved to 0.42 ± 0.15 after 2 years. Binocular vision improvement expressed by the proportion of patients who gained fusion and stereopsis was better overall in Group A (78%) than in Group B (33%). No complications were noted. The Authors conclude that PRK and LASEK are effective and safe methods for correcting high myopic anisometropia and improving amblyopia in 4-7 year old children who are CL intolerant. Visual acuity and binocular vision outcomes were better in children who received permanent surgical correction of anisometropia than in those who were treated conventionally by CLs.

In a similar study conducted by Tychsen et al[12], 36 eyes of 35 amblyopic children ( age range 4 to 16 years), received treatment for high ametropia. Seventy-two percent (25/35) of the children had a neurobehavioral disorder and/or were noncompliant with spectacle or contact lens wear. Myopia ranged from -3.25 to -24.25 D (mean, -11.48 D); one patient had hyperopia of +5.87 D. Correction was tailored to match the refractive error of the nonamblyopic eye and corneal centration was achieved using brief, general anesthesia. Mean follow-up was 29.2 months (range, 4-42 months). Eighty-nine percent (31 children) were corrected within ±1.00 D of target refraction and the remaining 11% to within ±2.0 D. Acuity improved postoperatively in 97%; by 1 line in 37% and by 2 or more lines in 60%. No child lost VA. Binocularity improved in 69% of patients and remained the same in 31%. Corneal haze was transitory and inversely proportional to patient age. Myopic regression occurred with a mean of 1.06 D/year. No substantial differences were observed in PRK versus LASEK treated children. The Authors suggest that keratocyte-mediated regrowth of the photoablated stroma and epithelial hyperplasia, toghether with axial growth, may be the main causes of myopic regression. Topical corticosteroids and systemic ascorbate (vitamin C) were used to reduce both stromal haze and regression.

Paysse et al[13], in a prospective study, treated with PRK 11 children, 2 to 11 years old, with anisometropic amblyopia who were noncompliant with conventional therapy with glasses or contact lenses and occlusion therapy. A cohort of 13 compliant and 10 noncompliant children with refractive errors similar to those of the PRK group who were treated with traditional anisometropic amblyopia therapy served as control groups. PRK was done on the eye with the higher refractive error.

Mean preoperative refractive errors were -13.70 ± 3.77 D for the myopic group and +4.75 ± 0.5 D for the hyperopic group. Mean postoperative refractive errors at last follow-up (mean, 31 months) were -3.5±2.25 D and +1.41 ± 1.07 D for the myopic and hyperopic groups, respectively. At the last follow-up, 63% of myopic children and 67% of hyperopic patients achieved a refraction within 2 D of the target refraction. Refractive regressions were 0.50 ± 1.41 (myopes) and 0.60 ± 0.57 D (hyperopes). Seven children (77%) were able to perform psychophysical VA testing preoperatively and postoperatively. Five (71%) of the 7 children had uncorrected VA improvement of at least 2 lines, and 4 (57%) of 7 had best spectacle-corrected VA improvement of at least 2 lines, with 1 improving 7 lines. Five (55%) of 9 children had improvement of their stereoacuity at last follow-up. Subepithelial corneal haze remained negligible. The mean final VA of the PRK group was significantly better than that of the noncompliant control group. The mean final refractive error for both myopic and hyperopic groups was also significantly better that that of the control.

The mean treatment decentration on the cornea of the 9 patients cooperative enough to undergo corneal topography was 0.68 mm. The child with the largest decentration was 7 years old at the time of the procedure and had a preoperative SE refractive error of 21.00 D with eccentric fixation.

Authors conclude that PRK seems to have potential as a treatment option for anisometropic amblyopia in children. The mild improvements in VA are justified by the fact the amblyopia was longstanding and severe. If anisometropia is treated at a younger age, amblyopia will likely be milder or may never even develop. Limit of this study is the small number of patients.

Amblyopia caused by anisometropia or bilateral refractive error, including astigmatism or nystagmus, often responds well to glasses if the amount of anisometropia is less than 3.00 D as indicated by Campos et al[14]. However, anisometropia greater than 1.50 D, especially myopic anisometropia, can induce dense amblyopia15. Because of the large amount of aniseikonia induced when refractive error is corrected, this form of amblyopia is especially resistant to more traditional forms of amblyopia therapy. However, with improvement in vision in the amblyopic eye, aniseikonia can become the most important factor in a child's inability to wear spectacle correction once amblyopia treatment is complete. Contact lenses are another option and provide better quality vision and a larger visual field with improved contrast sensitivity. However, full-time contact lens use by young children with coexisting ocular or medical problems is not always optimal or possible. These more complex anisometropic situations may be treated more effectively with laser refractive surgery.

In a retrospective study Astle et al[15] consider 53 children with anisometropia who had LASEK to correct the refractive difference between eyes after traditional methods of optical correction and amblyopia treatment were not successful. All LASEK procedures were performed under general anesthesia. Patients were divided into 3 groups according to their anisometropia as follows:myopic difference greater than 3.00 D, astigmatic difference greater than 1.50 D, and hyperopic difference greater than 3.50 D. The children were followed for at least 1 year, and their refractive status, visual acuity, and binocular vision were assessed and recorded at 2 and 6 months as well as 1 year. The mean age at treatment was 8.4 years (range 10 months to 16 years). The mean preoperative anisometropic difference was 6.98 D in the entire group, 9.48 D in the anisomyopic group, 3.13 D in the anisoastigmatic group, and 5.50 D in the anisohyperopic group. One year after LASEK, the mean anisometropic difference decreased to 1.81 D, 2.43 D, 0.74 D, and 2.33 D, respectively, and 54% of all eyes were within 1.00 D of the fellow eye. Postoperatively, 63.6% of children had an improvement in best corrected visual acuity (BCVA) and the remainder had no change. No patient had a reduction in BCVA or a loss in fusional ability after LASEK. Thirty nine percent had positive stereopsis preoperatively and 87.9% had positive stereopsis 1 year after LASEK. Authors suggest that elimination of the refractive component of the anisometropia provides major visual and functional improvement in children, with or without coexisting ocular and medical disorders.

Possible problems related to refractive surgery in children are topical anesthesia and lack of patient cooperation, the difficulty in obtaining treatment centration in general anesthesia due to absence of fixation, anatomical factors such as the higher risk of corneal ectasia, myopic shift and unforeseeable modifications due to eye growth[16]. No proven data exists on optimal correction of various refractive errors in order to prevent postoperative residual error or error progression due to eye growth or structural and morphologic corneal modifications[17].

Other possible problems include ocular alignment issues and increased ocular inflammatory responses like haze and uveitis. No data is published on possible postoperative endothelial damage, even if it is known that endothelium is more vulnerable in children.

## Hyperopia

In the last few years refractive surgery has been used for the correction of hyperopia and hyperopic astigmatism in children to prevent amblyopia, but limited data exists in literature when compared to laser treatment of myopic amblyopia.

Dvali et al[18] conducted a study on 63 eyes treated with LASIK over a 6 year period (46 patients, age range 8-16 yrs, mean age 12.65 yrs). No other form of amblyopia treatment was initiated during the study. Mean SE ranged from +1.0 to +6.0 D and astigmatism from 1.0 to 5.5 D. Mild to moderate amblyopia was present in 44 eyes, angle of deviation ranged from 10° to 45° in 30 patients and disruption of binocularity was seen in 24 cases. Follow up was 12 months. Preoperative UCVA ranged from 0.04 to 1.0, preoperative BSCVA ranged from 0.1 to 1.0. Postoperative UCVA ranged from 0.3 to 1.0, vision stabilized 3-6 months postoperatively. Postoperative UCVA was better than preoperative BSCVA in 70% of eyes. In this group degree of amblyopia decreased in 55% and disappeared in 45% of eyes. Angle of strabismus was significantly reduced or eliminated at 6 months. Twenty-one patients achieved binocularity. Authors conclude that laser correction of hyperopia and hyperopic astigmatism in children and adolescents has the potential to correct refractive errors, improve function in amblyopic eyes, correct accomodative strabismus and improve binocular vision.

This study has several limits. Precise information on the orthoptic examination and on previous antiamblyopic treatments is lacking, no information is given on the type of anesthesia or correlation of results with age or stability of results in the long term.

Yin et al[19] conducted a nonrandomized prospective study on 42 children with high hyperopic anisometropic amblyopia and 32 children with high myopic anisometropic amblyopia. All underwent LASIK to reduce their anisometropia. LASIK was performed under topical or general anesthesia. Follow-up ranged from 6 months to 3 years (average 17.45 months in the hyperopic group and 18.31 months in myopic group).

The mean preoperative binocular cycloplegic SE anisometropia was 6.13 ± 1.62 D (range, 3.50 to 7.75 D) in the hyperopic group and 10.13 ± 2.49 D (range, 15.75 to 5.37 D) in the myopic group. Hyperopic mean postoperative anisometropia was 0.56 ± 0.75 D at 3 years. Myopic mean postoperative anisometropia was 2.20 ± 1.05 D. The postoperative anisometropia was significantly reduced by the LASIK procedure in both groups.

The BCVA for distance and reading in the myopic group improved from 0.4 ± 0.25 and 0.58 ± 0.27, respectively, before surgery to 0.59 ± 0.28 and 0.96 ± 0.35, respectively, 3 years after surgery. In the hyperopic group BCVA for distance and reading improved from 0.23 ± 0.21 and 0.34 ± 0.32, respectively, before surgery to 0.53 ± 0.31 and 0.80 ± 0.33, respectively, 3 years after surgery. The proportion of patients who had stereopsis increased from 19.1% preoperatively to 46.7% postoperatively in the hyperopic group and from 19% to 89% in the myopic group.

The refractive stability was good in the hyperopic group up to 3 years postoperatively, no progressive hyperopic regression was found. Axial length remained stable throughout the 3 years of follow-up.

## Anesthesia

A variety of anesthetic techniques have been used for children undergoing refractive surgery. When possible, topical anesthesia is preferred over general anesthesia, because it allows the patient to self-fixate, reducing the likelihood of a decentered corneal ablation. In general, children older than 7 or 8 years of age seem to tolerate the procedure well under topical anesthesia. In some cases, premedication with an anxiolytic agent such as midazolam[20] or diazepam is added. Very young children usually require general anesthesia to ensure that the procedure is performed safely, especially in patients with neurobehavioural disorders.

A variety of agents, including nitrous oxide, sevoflurane, halothane, intravenous propofol[21], and intravenous ketamine[22], have been used to achieve general anesthesia. There is one report of nitrous oxide interfering with the laser, which resulted in the laser shutting off[23]. Because the wavelength of the Argon fluorine excimer beam is within the absorption spectrum of nitrous oxide, the nitrous oxide that escapes into the path of the excimer beam caused attenuation of the beam. This potential complication can averted by the anesthesiologist's performing the induction in an adjacent room or by the use of a laryngeal mask.

The limited longitudinal and lateral movements of the operating table and the position of the laser and the patient's head often don't allow proper ventilation and small spaces limit anesthesia procedures, postoperative monitoring and emergency procedures in case of serious complications[24,25].

For these reasons even if general anesthesia contributes to safety and efficacy of photoablation procedures, it is not free of complications, some of which serious and hard to handle without adequate facilities.

# Conclusions

Results are encouraging but further clinical studies with longer follow-up and larger series are needed.

# References

[1] Pediatric Eye Disease Investigator Group. Randomized trial of treatment of amblyopia in children aged 7 to 17 years. *Arch. Ophthalmol.* 2005; 123:437–447.

[2] Barequet IS, Wygnanski-Jaffe T, Hirsh A. Laser in situ keratomileusis improves visual acuity in some adult eyes with amblyopia. *J. Refract Surg.* 2004 Jan-Feb;20(1):25-8.

[3] Sakatani K, Jabbur NS, O'Brien TP. Improvement in best corrected visual acuity in amblyopic adult eyes after laser in situ keratomileusis. *J. Cataract Refract. Surg.* 2004 Dec;30(12):2517-21.

[4] Lanza M, Rosa N, Capasso L, Iaccarino G, Rossi S, Romano A. Can we utilize photorefractive keratectomy to improve visual acuity in adult amblyopic eyes? *Ophthalmology*. 2005 Oct;112(10):1684-91.

[5] El Mallah MK, Chakravarthy U, Hart PM. Amblyopia: is visual loss permanent? *Br. J. Ophthalmol.* 2000 Sep;84(9):952-6.

[6] Roszkowska AM, Biondi S, Chisari G, Messina A, Ferreri FM, Meduri A. Visual outcome after excimer laser refractive surgery in adult patients with amblyopia. *Eur. J. Ophthalmol.* 2006 Mar-Apr;16(2):214-8.

[7] France LW. Evidence based guidelines for amblyogenic risk factors. *Am. Orthopt. J.* 2006; 56:7–14

[8] Nucci P, Drack AV. Refractive surgery for unilateral high myopia in children. J AAPOS. 2001 Dec;5(6):348-51.

[9] Astle WF, Papp A, Huang PT, Ingram A. Refractive laser surgery in children with coexisting medical and ocular pathology. *J. Cataract Refract. Surg.* 2006 Jan;32(1):103-8.

[10] Astle WF, Huang PT, Ells AL, Cox RG, Deschenes MC, Vibert HM. Photorefractive keratectomy in children. *J. Cataract. Refract .Surg.* 2002 Jun;28(6):932-41.

[11] Autrata R, Rehurek J. Laser-assisted subepithelial keratectomy and photorefractive keratectomy versus conventional treatment of myopic anisometropic amblyopia in children. *J. Cataract. Refract .Surg.* 2004 Jan;30(1):74-84.

[12] Tychsen L, Packwood E, Berdy G. Correction of large amblyopiogenic refractive errors in children using the excimer laser. J AAPOS. 2005 Jun;9(3):224-33.

[13] Paysse EA, Coats DK, Hussein MA, Hamill MB, Koch DD. Long-term outcomes of photorefractive keratectomy for anisometropic amblyopia in children. *Ophthalmology*. 2006 Feb;113(2):169-76.

[14] Campos EC, Enoch JM. Amount of aniseikonia compatible with fine binocular vision: some old and new concepts. *J. Pediatr. Ophthalmol. Strabismus* 1980; 17:44-7.

[15] Astle WF, Rahmat J, Ingram AD, Huang PT. Laser-assisted subepithelial keratectomy for anisometropic amblyopia in children: outcomes at 1 year. *J. Cataract Refract. Surg.* 2007 Dec;33(12):2028-34.

[16] Braverman R. Diagnosis and treatment of refractive errors in the pediatric population. *Curr. Opin. Ophthalmol.* 2007 Sep;18(5):379-83.

[17] Moller-Pedersen T, Cavanagh HD, Petroll WM, Jester JV. Stromal wound healing explains refractive instability and haze development after photorefractive keratectomy: a 1-year confocal microscopic study. *Ophthalmology.* 2000 Jul;107(7):1235-45.

[18] Dvali ML, Tsintsadze NA, Mirtskhulava SI. Features of hyperopic LASIK in children. *J. Refract Surg.* 2005 Sep-Oct;21(5 Suppl):S614-6.

[19] Yin ZQ, Wang H, Yu T, Ren Q, Chen L. Facilitation of amblyopia management by laser in situ keratomileusis in high anisometropic hyperopic and myopic children. J AAPOS. 2007 Dec;11(6):571-6.

[20] Mahfouz AK, Khalaf MA. Comparative study of 2 anesthesia techniques for pediatric refractive surgery. *J. Cataract. Refract. Surg.* 2005 Dec;31(12):2345-9.

[21] Hertzog JH, Dalton HJ, Anderson BD, Shad AT, Gootenberg JE, Hauser GJ. Prospective evaluation of propofol anesthesia in the pediatric intensive care unit for elective oncology procedures in ambulatory and hospitalized children. *Pediatrics.* 2000 Oct;106(4):742-7.

[22] Oklü E, Bulutcu FS, Yalçin Y, Ozbek U, Cakali E, Bayindir O. Which anesthetic agent alters the hemodynamic status during pediatric catheterization? Comparison of propofol versus ketamine. *.J Cardiothorac. Vasc. Anesth.* 2003 Dec;17(6):686-90.

[23] Cook DR, Dhaliwal DK, Davis PJ, Davis J. Anesthetic interference with laser function during excimer laser procedures in children. Anesth Analg. 2001 Jun;92(6):1444-5.

[24] Mazurek MS. Sedation and analgesia for procedures outside the operating room. Semin. Pediatr. Surg. 2004 Aug;13(3):166-73.

[25] Yldzdaş D, Yapcoglu H, Ylmaz HL. The value of capnography during sedation or sedation/analgesia in pediatric minor procedures. Pediatr Emerg. Care. 2004 Mar;20(3):162-5.

In: Laser Keratectomy: Approaches, Complications... ISBN 978-1-60456-863-9
Author: Luis W. Schröder and Felix J. Walter 

*Chapter VIII*

# The New Era of Refractive Correction

***Marco Lombardo*** **[*]** ***and Giuseppe Lombardo***
Vision Engineering, Rome and Reggio Calabria, Italy
INFM-CNR LiCryL Laboratory, Physics Department, University of Calabria, Arcavacata di Rende (CS), Italy

## Abstract

During the last decade, advances in the knowledge and measurement of the eye's optical aberrations have moved the wave aberration theory from an obscure scientific concept to one that is central to efforts to improve vision. Nowadays, all the imperfections in the components and materials within the eye that cause light rays to deviate from the desired path are referred to as *optical aberrations*. Refractive surgery aims to minimize optical aberrations in the eye. Excimer laser surgery is the most performed surgical technique to improve unaided vision. The personalized correction of the eye's aberrations promises to be the next golden standard in laser refractive surgery. The technique necessitates an accurate determination of the wavefront error and a precise system of surgical correction. To date, although it has been demonstrated that image quality after customized procedures is improved over that of standard procedures, there are still significant aberrations induced after a wavefront-guided procedure that are neither expected nor predicted. The ability to anticipate confounding biophysical responses of the cornea at the level of the individual patient remains still limited and should be improved.

The development of innovative wavefront sensing and correcting methods and techniques is now opening new perspectives of high-precision refractive corrections. Data coming from the reliable measurements of the corneal and ocular wave aberration may be used to drive a more precise personalized correction of the eye's aberrations for eliminating low-order aberrations and further compensating high-order aberrations between cornea and lens to optimize the individual visual performance. Accordingly, identifying all the components of corneal biophysical response to develop therapeutic

[*] Address correspondence to: Dr. Marco Lombardo, MD, PhD, via Adda, 7 – 00198, Rome – ITALY, Phone and Fax: +39 06 88 40 971, E-mail: mlombardo@visioeng.it

models for compensating for these factors will ultimately lead to increased predictability of visual outcomes.

Major advances in presbyopia correction are also expected in the near future, thanks to the application of innovative electro-optical technologies, such as liquid crystals, in vision science.

# Expert Commentary

## Causes and Sources of Vision Blurring

Vision begins with the formation of an optical image of the external world upon the retinal mosaic of light-sensitive photoreceptors. Because image formation is the very first step in the visual process, imperfections in the eye's optical apparatus have the potential for affecting every aspect of visual perception. The eye is an optical system having several optical elements for focusing light rays representing images onto the retina. Imperfections in the components and materials within the eye may cause light rays to deviate from the desired path. These deviations, referred to as *optical aberrations*, result in blurred images and decreased visual performance. Optical aberrations from the eye include low-order and high-order aberrations. Low-order aberrations, i.e., defocus and astigmatism, are the predominant optical aberrations in the human eye: they account for 90% to the overall wave aberration (WA) of the eye and are currently well corrected with spectacles, contact lenses or laser surgery. Although high-order aberrations (HOA) make a small contribution (≤10%) to the total variance of the eye wave aberration, their correction improves visual performance substantially, as largely demonstrated with the use of Adaptive Optics techniques [1]. An increasing number of studies has shown the deleterious effect of HOA on image quality [2,3], especially for larger pupil sizes. On the other hand, HOA cannot be corrected adequately with current mainstream optical or surgical treatments. How HOA decrease the human visual performance is currently subject of debate [4]. The Rayleigh and Maréchal criterions [5] suggest that if the ocular WA exceeded a quarter-wavelength ($\lambda/4$: about 0.14 microns for green light) the image would be significantly degraded with respect to the diffraction-limited case [6]. Ocular and corneal wavefront sensors are capable of measuring with extreme precision sub-wavelength errors of the eye optics and we are already aware that the ocular wavefront typically exceeds this quarter-wave limit [7]. Hence, it is reasonable to expect that the full correction of the eye's WA will almost definitely lead to significant improvements in optical image quality. Authors reported that an aberration-minimizing procedure has to provide an ablation depth per pulse lower than 0.1 μm [8]. This calculation indicates that present day laser devices that work with an ablation rate of 0.25 μm per pulse may be improved; however, it is probable that wound healing and biomechanical effects may limit the precision of laser corneal reshaping [9,10].

Beyond optical aberrations, the human eye suffers also from *scattering*, *dispersion* of light and *diffraction*. *Scattering* occurs whenever light encounters refractive index discontinuities in its path. *Scatter* in the ocular media is mainly due to diffusion and the loss of transparency in the cornea, the lens, and the humours. The result of *dispersion* of the light in optical elements of the eye is the induction of chromatic aberrations. In other words, chromatic aberration is simply spherical refractive error that depends on wavelength. *Diffraction* is a fundamental property of the wave nature of light whenever it passes through the eye and the edge of the iris [11]. In theory, it is possible to improve image quality in the eye by reducing aberrations, but it is impossible to exceed the limits to image quality set by the unavoidable optical imperfections within the eye, such as scattering, dispersion or, most of all, diffraction. Ultimate optical quality is therefore referred to as "diffraction limited", that is, limited by diffraction only. Without aberrations, the perfect eye would convert incoming wavefronts into converging spherical waves. Thus, the effect of diffraction is to cause the image of a point to have a finite size: this point image resulting from diffraction is called the *Airy disk*.

During the past decade, there has been a remarkable expansion of the application of wavefront-related technologies to human eyes. Methods for measuring the optical aberrations of the individual eye have made possible large population ocular wavefront analysis. It is now well known that the form of the ocular WA varies substantially with the individual, presumably depending upon the surface asymmetries and surface tilts between the optical components of the particular eye and their relative locations with respect to the pupil. Various studies [3,7,12] have measured the distribution and contribution of each high-order aberration to the overall wavefront aberration of the eye, showing how there is a central tendency for human eyes to be free of higher-order aberrations, but with the individual aberration equally likely to have positive or negative value because of random biological variability. The one clear exception among the higher-order modes is spherical aberration which is systematically biased towards positive values. Also, there is no clear evidence that aberrations vary systematically with degree of ametropia [13]. The only distinction between eyes is that astigmatic eyes tend to have slightly larger total amount of higher-order aberrations than myopic, hyperopic or emmetropic eyes.

The optical performance of the normal eye is governed by the combination of aberrations in the corneal and intra-ocular optics and it has been shown that there is a significant correlation between these elements [14,15]. Different studies [16,17,18] have measured that the total amount of the WA for the whole eye is always less than values for either the anterior cornea or the internal optics. The results are explained by compensatory processing between the cornea and the lens. However, the compensation observed in young eyes is not present for older subjects and this has been related to a decrease in visual performance with aging [19,20].

Particular attention has also been devoted to the interocular balance of optical aberrations in order to better characterize binocular visual performance. Recent works [21,22,23,24,25,26] have demonstrated a mirror symmetry of the high-order WA maps of the cornea as well as the whole eye optics between eyes, especially for third and fourth order terms over a dilated pupil. It is also well known that the eye's wave aberration is not static but fluctuates over time. The largest source of temporal short-term instability (seconds and minutes) is micro-fluctuations in accommodation. Other possible causes for the fluctuations include local changes in tear film thickness over the cornea [27], perhaps caused by evaporation or blinking. On the other hand, the eye's WA has been demonstrated to be sufficiently stable over long periods of time (over the course of the day, and between successive days), indicating that a personalized aberration correction would be valuable.

Thanks to the increased longevity of people, the effect of aging on HOA of the human eye has also been largely investigated [28,29,30,31,32]. It has been reported that the amount of corneal and ocular HOA increases approximately linearly with age with a corresponding decline in visual performance [33,34]. The spherical aberration has been found on average to be slightly larger in older corneas, as also coma and other corneal HOA that showed to increase with aging. The increase in spherical aberration has been mainly related to a change in the asphericity of the cornea, which occurs from younger to older subjects. The overall shape of the cornea tends to become a sphere from an ellipsoid as age increases. As specified above, the net result of the decoupling of aberrations between the cornea and the internal eye optics is a decrease in visual performance. This is an important issue as it relates all the people that undergo to corneal laser ablation, where the decoupling of aberrations between eye optics is induced by the surgery itself [35].

Nowadays, presbyopia represents a major visual impairment of aging, due to the decline of lens ability to focus on near distance objects after age 45. The mechanism by which the eye can change focus on near and distant objects or *accommodation* has been debated for long centuries. The Helmholtz theory [36] indicates the impossibility of obtaining a variation in curvature of the crystalline lens following atrophy of the ciliary muscle. The Schachar theory [37] states that presbyopia is due to a decrease in the effective working distance of the ciliary muscle as a result of a normal increase in equatorial volume of the crystalline lens with aging.

The acquired knowledge of the aberration architecture of human eyes has generated an intensive effort to revise methods and techniques to correct vision. Novel technologies of measuring and correcting optical aberrations, have offered the promise of a new generation of vision correction methods that can correct HOA beyond defocus and astigmatism, enhancing visual performance beyond that provided by current treatments.

## Wavefront Sensing and Correcting Techniques

The evolution of the field of wavefront sensing has proceeded at an extremely rapid pace since initially conceived. Nowadays, various wavefront sensing techniques have been developed for the measurement of the eye's WA. In general, all the apparatus include a source for generating the beam for producing the wavefront exiting the eye, a sensor element and an imaging device for receiving the wavefront to determine aberrations. Wavefront sensors measure the aberrations of the entire eye generated both by the corneal surface and the crystalline lens (*ocular aberrometer*), whereas corneal topographer can measure only the aberrations induced by the first corneal surface (*corneal aberrometer*).

The Shack-Hartmann (S-H) wavefront sensor [38] is the most employed technique for measuring the optical quality of the eye. The device was introduced in clinical use in the 1990s. This technique has been used in several areas of clinical research, e.g., studies of myopia, dry eye, keratoconus, cataract, refractive surgery, contact lenses and intraocular lenses [39,40,41,42], giving initial results on the wave aberration distribution in normal and diseased eye populations. On the other hand, the limited *dynamic range* and *measurement sensitivity* of this technique posed the basis for research efforts to design and develop alternative and innovative wavefront sensing techniques. Between these, curvature sensing [43], pyramidal sensing [44] and interferometry [45] are the most studied techniques to overcome the major disadvantages of the S-H sensor: they can achieve a larger dynamic range providing high accuracy measurements even in highly aberrated eyes. A more reliable estimation of the eye's optical aberrations will be valuable for different applications, such as the personalization of laser refractive surgery or the fabrication of personalized contact lenses and intra-ocular lenses. In addition, such an accurate wavefront sensor may represent a key element to develop a reliable and fast Adaptive Optics system for clinical purpose [46].

Adaptive Optics (AO) is a technique developed in astronomy to remove the effect of atmospheric turbulence from telescope image. The success of AO in astronomy and the declassification of the military's information in 1992, stimulated progress for other applications, including Ophthalmology.

AO can, in principle, correct for the total WA of the eye by altering the local optical path at each point in the pupil by an appropriate amount so that the overall paths for rays entering all points in the pupil are equal. Moreover, AO allows to perform experiments to better understand the impact of ocular optics on vision and in particular to explore the possible role of the neural system in sharpening the retinal images. Some experiments have indicated that not every aberration will have the same impact on vision [14] and how corneal and intraocular optics can interact to modulate visual performance in different light conditions [15,16]. Accordingly, an AO system can be used as a visual simulator to test in advance the effect of aberration correction produced by refractive surgery. Nowadays, deformable mirrors are the most popular devices for AO [46,47]. Former experiments revealed how this technology is effective in achieving a controllable and accurate measurement and correction of ocular aberrations [48,49]. On the other hand, there are many reasons to search for alternative solutions for application of AO in the clinical environment. The relative cost and dimension of this technology represent a major limitation for a wider use other than in laboratory. Therefore, many researchers in the world are studying and applying different AO methodologies to get this technology compact, relatively low-cost and effective for the every day clinical practice. To do this, different issues, as noise, speckle, error propagation and the dynamics of ocular aberrations, have to be studied and understood. The cumulative research work over the last few years is beginning to provide enough data to improve our understanding of most of these issues. Recently, new technologies for wavefront correction have been developed based on microelectromechanical mirrors (MEMM) [50,51,52] and liquid crystal spatial light modulators (LC-SLM) [53,54], which are both successful at reducing the WA of the eye and less expensive than conventional DM devices. The compactness of these new solutions and the continuous improvement in resolution and performance of these correcting elements justify the forecast of prospective clinical applications of AO technology.

## The Present of Refractive Correction

Most of refractive surgery procedures involve altering the cornea; between these the excimer laser corneal surgery is the most commonly performed procedure for correcting myopia, hyperopia and astigmatism. Photorefractive keratectomy (PRK) [55] was the first technique performed; subsequently, laser in situ keratomileusis (LASIK) has become largely popular to correct the refractive defects of the eye. Other laser techniques include laser epithelial keratomileusis (LASEK) [56] and Epi-Lasik [57].

There are, however, various keratorefractive procedures to correct for refractive errors, such as the insertion of intrastromal corneal ring segments, the removal of clear crystalline lens, the implantation of phakic intraocular lens and conductive keratoplasty. These techniques are much less performed than excimer laser surgery, due to the less predictability of results; on the other hand, they may be preferred in particular cases. The intracorneal ring segment (ICRS) procedure involves placing plastic arcuate segments into channels created in the stroma of the midperipheral cornea. The central corneal shape is altered by the configuration of the segments and their location in the cornea. The application of this procedure is very limited due to its complications and lack of results. Currently, ICRS has been applied to reduce the irregular astigmatism of keratoconus [58]. Removal of the clear crystalline lens, with or without intra-ocular lens (IOL) implantation, has been performed to correct high hyperopic or myopic refractive errors for many years. Also, specially designed IOLs may be surgically placed in the anterior chamber, attached to the iris [59], or placed in the posterior chamber anterior to the crystalline lens [60] in the phakic eye to correct high myopic or hyperopic refractive errors. Conductive keratoplasty (CK) is performed to correct for hyperopia or presbyopia [61]; it uses a contact probe to deliver radio frequency energy by inserting the thin insulated tip sequentially in multiple locations of the peripheral cornea. The energy produces shrinkage of collagen lamellae that leads to steepening of the central cornea. The amount of change depends on a number of variables including the total amount of energy delivered, number of pulses, pulse energy, spot size, and clear zone, showing a moderate variability of refractive outcomes in the long term postoperative period [62].

Besides CK, the correction of presbyopia include other surgical methods or techniques, such as monovision, multifocal photoablation, anterior ciliary sclerotomy (ACS), scleral expansion bands, multifocal or accommodating IOLs, and intracorneal inlays. At present, the most widely used surgical approach to compensate for presbyopia is excimer laser photoablation to create monovision or inducing a different HOA architecture in the cornea by means of inferior off-center ablation or multifocal ablation [63, 64]. ACS [65] has been largely abandoned due to lack of efficacy and complications such as anterior segment ischemia, regression, and lack of effect. Scleral expansion bands [66] are currently being investigated as a means of increasing the distance between the ciliary muscle and lens.

Early results of accommodating and zonal-progressive multifocal [67,68] IOLs have been shown to reduce presbyopic symptoms. On the other hand, drawbacks included a progressive efficacy reduction in the years following surgery, increased glare and some reduction in low-contrast visual acuity.

## The Future of Refractive Correction

During the last decade, photorefractive surgery has dramatically evolved with the simultaneous development of more precise laser platforms and systems for measuring the optical properties of the individual eye. The accurate analysis of new corneal topographer and ocular wavefront sensors has revealed that although standard laser refractive surgery eliminates conventional refractive errors, high-order errors are typically induced [35,40]. The dynamic evaluation of optical quality performed by AO systems has also revealed the effect of aberrations on visual performance [2].

The success of aberration-related techniques encourages the implementation of high-order correction in everyday vision through customized laser refractive surgery or also contact or intraocular lenses. The use of a reliable wavefront sensor capable to measure the whole eye optical aberrations, integrated with the data coming from videokeratoscopes [69], can refine algorithms of current excimer laser systems in order to achieve accurate ablation of the individual cornea. The personalization of the corneal ablation may be achieved transferring data output from the wavefront sensor and corneal topographer/aberrometer to the laser platform; the cornea will be accordingly remodeled for eliminating low-order aberrations and compensating high-order aberrations between the cornea and lens in order to optimize the visual performance for the individual. To reach the scope, future algorithms should take into account the predicted biomechanical response of the cornea based on individual geometrical features of the tissue.

Current excimer laser devices are capable to remove infinitesimally amount of corneal tissue (i.e., 0.25 μm), however, some inaccuracies, like the ablation profile and parameters as well as the biophysical response of the cornea, still limit the potential visual benefit one could achieve from reshaping the cornea [70]. Many authors are analyzing the possible predictors of individual responses [10,71,72] in order to develop accurate models for controlling or compensating for the biophysical responses of the corneal tissue to surgery [73]. The aim of research in this setting is, therefore, strictly linked to advancements in laser platform ablation parameters to improve visual outcomes of laser refractive surgery. Laser manufacturers are currently investigating ways to either minimize or compensate for the corneal biomechanical response as suggested by clinical researchers. The fundamental Munnerlyn theory [55] stating that the cornea is an homogeneous inert structure has been extensively demonstrated not to be adequate for modeling the behaviour of the corneal tissue. Since 1995, when a biomechanical response of the cornea after laser ablation has been first hypothesized [74], several models based on empirical analyses of postoperative data and on more complex assumptions on the corneal behaviour have been developed [75,76,77,78, 79]. The scope of these researches was to improve the predictability of results, further optimizing the postoperative optical quality of the cornea. The new question raising from recent studies is whether the biomechanical response can be manipulated to improve outcomes. For instance, clinical studies have demonstrated a mirror symmetric response of the anterior cornea to laser ablation, with the nasal peripheral region straining more than the temporal, and also a different response of the corneal periphery in relation to the amount of refractive correction [72,80]. The target of these studies was to drive the design of ablation profiles, by modifying the transition zone, in order to compensate for the invariable part of the corneal response. Further refinements in the ablation design should be then performed to optimize the procedure, depending on the geometrical and optical parameters of the individual cornea. These personalized improved algorithms can be, for instance, developed by analysing topographic and aberrometric data in a large population of eyes prior and after laser reshaping.

Moreover, wavefront sensing and correcting technologies can be further exploited to drive the fabrication of personalized contact lenses (CLs) or intraocular lenses (IOLs) by transferring the data output of the eye's WA to the manufacturing instruments. Recent advances in intraocular lens materials and manufacturing methods [81] make the customized correction of higher-order aberrations with CLs or IOLs to become standard practice in the next years [82].

In the context of customized refractive correction, new ideas for near-vision correction are expected. Considering that the replacement of cataractous crystalline lens with accommodating or pseudo-accommodating IOLs and other surgical solutions for the correction of presbyopia appear not to be effective in restoring adequate near vision performance, the research in this setting has not still shown significant advancements. Restoring accommodation represents the golden target of future refractive correction methods if considering that an incredible number of people worldwide need to wear spectacles for near vision.

The application of innovative technologies in Ophthalmology, such as liquid crystals, to replace common lenses to deviate light rays aims to solve and overcome limits of current methodologies for improving near vision in elderly population. During the last years, innovative researches are going to demonstrate the way to replace common lenses for vision correction with *variable lenses* exploiting the liquid crystal (LC) technology [83,84]. A research area is directed to develop a switchable, flat, liquid-crystal diffractive lens that can adaptively change its focusing power to correct for distance and near vision. A different area involves the development of an adaptive intraocular lens based on a modal liquid-crystal spatial phase modulator with wireless control. A prototype has been developed and experimentally evaluated [85]. The goal of these studies is to provide a controllable IOL with variable focusing power. Even if a not pure LC lens may be achieved but rather a sort of hybrid lens in which ordinary glass is used to correct the sphero-cylindrical refractive error and the liquid crystal display is used to correct the residual, higher order aberrations, we believe that both solutions have the potential of revolutionizing the field of presbyopia correction in the near future. Therefore, the LC technology appears to have the potential for providing an entirely new kind of electro-optical elements for 21$^{st}$ century spectacles or intra-ocular lenses.

# Conclusion

In summary, we forecast major advances in vision correction treatments in the near future which will combine the power of wavefront-related technologies with the flexibility of electronics. The result will be a new generation of personalized laser treatment and variable spectacles or intra-ocular lenses capable of adapting to the specific requirements of individual eyes to produce customized optical correction of unprecedented quality. However, to make this prediction come true will require joint research efforts between the ophthalmic and engineering communities to apply these innovative technologies in the every day clinical practice.

## References

[1] Porter J, Guirao A, Cox IG, Williams DR. Monochromatic aberrations of the human eye in a large population. *J. Opt. Soc. Am. A*, 2001, 18, 1793-1803.

[2] Williams DR, Yoon G-Y, Porter J, Guirao A, Hofer H, Cox I. Visual benefit of correcting higher order aberrations of the eye. *J. Refract. Surg.*, 2000, 16, S554-S559.

[3] Thibos LN, Hong X, Bradley A, Cheng X. Statistical variation of aberration structure and image quality in a normal population of healthy eyes. *J. Opt. Soc. Am. A*, 2002, 19, 2329-2348.

[4] Applegate RA, Marsack JD, Ramos R, Sarver EJ. Interaction between aberrations to improve or reduce visual performance. *J. Cataract Refract. Surg.*, 2003, 29, 1487-1495.

[5] Rayleigh Lord. Encyclopaedia Britannica, Vol.8, New York, 245, 1910.

[6] Charman WN, Chateau N. The prospects for super-acuity: limits to visual performance after correction of monochromatic ocular aberration. *Ophthal. Physiol. Opt.*, 2003, 23, 479-493.

[7] Porter J, Guirao A, Cox IG, Williams DA. The human eye's monochromatic aberrations in a large population, *J. Opt. Soc. Am. A*, 2001, 18, 1793-1803.

[8] Manns F, Ho A, Parel JM, Culbertson W. Ablation profiles for wavefront-guided correction of myopia and primary spherical aberration, *J. Cataract Refract. Surg.*, 2002, 28, 766-774.

[9] Netto MV, Mohan RR, Ambrosio R, Hutcheon AEK, Zieske JD, Wilson SE. Wound Healing in the Cornea. A Review of Refractive Surgery Complications and New Prospects for Therapy. *Cornea,* 2005, 24, 509–522.

[10] Dupps WJ, Wilson SE. Biomechanics and wound healing in the cornea. *Exp. Eye Res.,* 2006, 83, 709-720.

[11] Born M, Wolf E. Principles of Optics; Electromagnetic theory of propagation, interference and diffraction of light. New York, Pergamon Press, 1975.

[12] Thibos LN, Bradley A, Hong X. A statistical model of the aberration structure of normal, well-corrected eyes. *Ophthal. Physiol. Opt.*, 2002, 22, 427-433.

[13] Cheng X, Bradley A, Hong X, Thibos LN. Relationship between refractive error and monochromatic aberrations of the eye. *Optom. Vis. Sci.*, 2003, 80, 43-49.

[14] Applegate RA, Marsack JD, Ramos R, Sarver EJ. Interaction between aberrations to improve or reduce visual performance. *J. Cataract Refract. Surg.*, 2003, 29, 1487-1495.

[15] Mrochen M, Jankov M, Bueeler M, Seiler T. Correlation between corneal and total wavefront aberrations in myopic eyes. *J. Refract. Surg.*, 2003, 19, 104-112.

[16] Artal P, Guirao A, Berrio E, Williams DR. Compensation of corneal aberrations by the internal optics in the human eye. *J. Vision*, 2001, 1, 1-8.

[17] Artal P, Guirao A, Berrio E, Piers P. Contribution of the cornea and internal surfaces to the change of ocular aberrations with age. *J. Opt. Soc. Am. A*, 2002, 19, 137-143.

[18] He JC, Gwiazda J, Thorn F, Held R. Wave-front aberrations in the anterior corneal surface and the whole eye. *J. Opt. Soc. Am. A*, 2003, 20, 1155-1163.

[19] Marcos S. Are changes in ocular aberrations with age a significant problem for refractive surgery? *J. Refract. Surg.*, 2002, 18, S572-S578.

[20] Guirao A, Gonzalez C, Redondo M, Geraghty E, Norrby S, Artal P. Average optical performance of the human eye as a function of age in a normal population. *Invest. Ophthalmol. Vis. Sci.*, 1999, 40, 203-213.

[21] Bogan SJ, Waring III GO, Ibrahim O, Drews C, Curtis L. Classification of normal corneal topography based on computer-assisted videokeratography. *Arch. Ophthalmol.*, 1990, 108, 945-949.

[22] Myrowitz EH, Kouzis AC, O'Brien TP. High interocular corneal symmetry in average simulated keratometry, central corneal thickness, and posterior elevation. *Optom. Vis. Sci.*, 2005, 82, 428-431.

[23] Liu Z, Huang AJ, Pflugfelder SC. Evaluation of corneal thickness and topography in normal eyes using the Orbscan corneal topography system. *Br. J. Ophthalmol.*, 1999, 83, 774-778.

[24] Wang L, Koch DD. Ocular higher-order aberrations in individuals screened for refractive surgery. *J. Cataract Refract. Surg.*, 2003, 29, 1896-1903.

[25] Castejon-Mochón JF, López-Gil N, Benito A, Artal P. Ocular wave-front aberration statistics in a normal young population. *Vision Res.*, 2002, 42, 1611-1617.

[26] Lombardo M, Lombardo G, Serrao S. Interocular high-order corneal wavefront aberration symmetry. *J. Opt. Soc. Am. A*, 2006, 23, 777-787.

[27] Thibos LN. The prospects for perfect vision. *J. Refract. Surg.*, 2000, 16, S540-S546.

[28] Calver RI, Cox MJ, Elliot DB. Effect of aging on the monochromatic aberrations of the human eye. *J. Opt. Soc. Am. A*, 1999, 16, 2069-2078.

[29] Guirao A, Redondo M, Artal P. Optical aberrations of the human cornea as a function of age. *J. Opt. Soc. Am. A*, 2000, 17, 1697-1702.

[30] Fujikado T, Kuroda T, Ninomiya S, Maeda N, Tano Y, Oshika T, Hirohara Y, Mihashi T. Age-related changes in ocular and corneal aberrations. *Am. J. Ophthalmol.*, 2004, 138, 143-146.

[31] Amano S, Amano Y, Yamagami S, Miyai T, Miyata K, Samejima T, Oshika T. Age-related changes in corneal and ocular higher-order wavefront aberrations. *Am. J. Ophthalmol.*, 2004, 137, 988-992.

[32] Kuroda T, Fujikado T, Ninomiya S, Maeda N, Hirohara Y, Mihashi T. Effect of aging on ocular light scatter and higher order aberrations. *J. Refract. Surg.*, 2002, 18, S598-S602.

[33] Oshika T, Klyce SD, Applegate RA, Howland HC. Changes in corneal wavefront aberrations with aging. *Invest. Ophthalmol. Vis. Sci.*, 1999, 40, 1351-1355.

[34] Shahidi M, Yang Y. Measurements of ocular aberrations and light scatter in healthy subjects. *Optom. Vis. Sci.*, 2004, 81, 853-857.

[35] Lombardo M, Lombardo G, Serrao S. Long-term optical quality of the photoablated cornea. *J. Opt. Soc. Am. A*, 2007, 24, 588-596.

[36] Von Helmholtz H. Treatise on Physiological Optics, 3rd ed. JPCt Southall (Washington, 1909, English translation by Optical Society of America 1924).

[37] Schachar RA, Cudmore DP, Black TD. Experimental support for Schachar's hypothesis of accommodation. *Ann. Ophthalmol.* 1993; 25: 404-409.

[38] Platt R, Shack R. History and principles of Shack-Hartmann wavefront sensing. *J. Refract. Surg.*, 2001, 17, S573-S577.

[39] Thibos LN, Hong X. Clinical applications of the Shack-Hartmann aberrometer. *Optom. Vis. Sci.*, 1999, 76, 817-825.

[40] Miller JM, Anwaruddin R, Straub J, Schwiegerling J. Higher order aberrations in normal, dilated, intraocular lens, and laser in situ keratomileusis corneas. *J. Refract. Surg.*, 2002, 18, S579-S583.

[41] Kuroda T, Fujikado T, Maeda N, Oshika T, Hirohara Y, Mihashi T. Wavefront analysis of higher-order aberrations in patients with cataract. *J. Cataract Refract. Surg.*, 2002, 28, 438–44.

[42] Marsack J, Milner T, Rylander G, Leach N, Roorda A. Applying wavefront sensors and corneal topography to keratoconus. *Biomed. Sci. Instrum.*, 2002, 38, 471–476.

[43] Diaz-Douton F, Pujol J, Arjona M, Luque SO. Curvature sensor for ocular wavefront measurement. *Opt. Lett.*, 2006, 31, 2245-2247.

[44] Chamot SR, Dainty C, Esposito S. Adaptive optics for ophthalmic applications using a pyramid wavefront sensor. *Opt. Exp.*, 2006, 2, 518-526.

[45] Shirai T, Barnes TH. Adaptive restoration of a partially coherent blurred image using an all-optical feedback interferometer with a liquid-crystal device. *J. Opt. Soc. Am. A*, 2002, 19, 369-377.

[46] Porter J, Queener H, Lin J, Thorn K, Awwal A. Adaptive optics for vision science; I Ed.; Hoboken, NJ, USA; John Wiley & Sons, Inc.; 2006.

[47] Liang J, Williams DR, Miller DT. Supernormal vision and high-resolution retinal imaging through adaptive optics. *J. Opt. Soc. Am. A*, 1997, 14, 2884-2892.

[48] Fernandez EJ, Iglesias I, Artal P. Closed-loop adaptive optics in the human eye. *Opt. Lett.*, 2001, 26, 746–748.

[49] Hofer H, Chen L, Yoon GY, Singer B, Yamauchi Y, Williams DR. Improvement in retinal image quality with dynamic correction of the eye's aberrations. *Opt. Expr.*, 2001, 8, 631-643.

[50] Doble N, Yoon G, Chen L. The use of a microelectromechanical mirror for adaptive optics in the human eye. *Opt. Lett.*, 2002, 27, 1537-1539.

[51] Fernandez EJ, Artal P. Membrane deformable mirror for adaptive optics: performance limits in visual optics. *Opt. Expr.*, 2003, 11, 1056-1069.

[52] Zhang Y, Poonja S, Roorda A. MEMS-based adaptive optics scanning laser ophthalmoscopy. *Opt. Lett.*, 2006, 31, 1268-1270.

[53] Prieto PM, Fernandez EJ, Manzanera S, Artal P. Adaptive optics with a programmable phase modulator: applications in the human eye. *Opt. Expr.*, 2004, 12, 4059-4071.

[54] Fernandez EJ, Považai B, Hermann, Unterhuber A, Sattmann H, Prieto PM, Leitgeb R, Ahneit P, Artal P, Drexler W. Three-dimensional adaptive optics ultra-high resolution optical coherence tomography using a liquid crystal spatial light modulator. *Vis. Res.*, 2005, 45, 3432-3444.

[55] Munnerlyn CR, Koons SJ, Marshall J. Photorefractive keratectomy: a technique for laser refractive surgery. *J. Cataract Refract. Surg.*, 1988,14, 46-52.

[56] Taneri S, Zieske JD, Azar DT. Evolution, techniques, clinical outcomes, and pathophysiology of LASEK: review of the literature. *Surv. Ophthalmol.*, 2004, 49, 576-602.

[57] Pallikaris IG, Katsanevaki V.J., Kalyvianaki MI, Naoumidi II. Advances in subepithelial excimer refractive surgery techniques: Epi-LASIK. *Curr. Opin. Ophthalmol.*, 2003, 14, 207-212.

[58] Alió JL, Shabayek MH, Artola A. Intracorneal ring segments for keratoconus correction: long-term follow-up. *J. Cataract Refract. Surg.*, 2006, 32, 978-985.

[59] Moshirfar M, Holz HA, Davis DK. Two-year follow-up of the Artisan/Verisyse iris-supported phakic intraocular lens for the correction of high myopia. *J. Cataract Refract. Surg.*, 2007, 33, 1392-1397.

[60] Tsiklis NS, Kymionis GD, Karp CL, Naoumidi T, Pallikaris AI. Nine-year follow-up of a posterior chamber phakic IOL in one eye and LASIK in the fellow eye of the same patient. *J. Refract. Surg.*, 2007, 23, 935-937.

[61] Stahl JE. Conductive keratoplasty for presbyopia: 3-year results. *J. Refract. Surg.*, 2007, 23, 905-910.

[62] Pallikaris IG, Naoumidi TL, Astyrakakis NI. Long-term results of conductive keratoplasty for low to moderate hyperopia. *J. Cataract Refract. Surg.*, 2005, 31, 1520-1529.

[63] Baueberg JM. Centered vs. inferior off-center ablation to correct hyperopia and presbyopia. *J. Refract. Surg.*, 1999, 15, 66-69.

[64] Telandro A. Pseudo-accomodative cornea: a new concept for correction of presbyopia. *J. Refract. Surg.*, 2004, 20, S714-S717.

[65] Hamilton DR, Davidorf JM, Maloney RK. Anterior ciliary sclerotomy for treatment of presbyopia: a prospective controlled study. *Ophthalmology,* 2002, 109, 1970-1976.

[66] Malecaze FJ, Gazagne CS, Tarroux MC, Gorrand JM. Scleral expansion bands for presbyopia. *Ophthalmology,* 2001, 108, 2165-2171.

[67] Uthoff D, Gulati A, Hepper D, Holland D. Potentially accommodating 1CU intraocular lens: 1-year results in 553 eyes and literature review. *J. Refract. Surg.,* 2007, 23, 159-171.

[68] Pepose JS, Qazi MA, Davies J, Doane JF, Loden JC, Sivalingham V, Mahmoud AM. Visual performance of patients with bilateral vs combination Crystalens, ReZoom, and ReSTOR intraocular lens implants. *Am. J. Ophthalmol.,* 2007, 144, 347-357.

[69] Mrochen M, Jankov M, Bueeler M, Seiler T. Correlation between corneal and total wavefront aberrations in myopic eyes. *J. Refract. Surg.*, 2003, 19, 104-112.

[70] Lombardo M, Lombardo G, De Santo MP, Barberi R, Serrao S. Roughness of excimer laser ablated corneas with and without smoothing measured with atomic force microscopy. *J. Refract. Surg.*, 2005, 21, 469-475.

[71] Roberts C. The cornea is not a piece of plastic. *J. Refract. Surg.,* 2000, 16, 407-413.

[72] Lombardo M, Lombardo G, Manzulli M, Serrao S. Response of the cornea for up to four-years after photorefractive keratectomy. *J. Refract. Surg*., 2006, 22, 178-186.

[73] Djotyan GP, Kurtz RM, Fernández DC, Juhasz T. An analytically solvable model for biomechanical response of the cornea to refractive surgery. *J. Biomech. Eng.*, 2001, 123, 440-445.

[74] Dupps WJ, Roberts C, Schoessler JP. Peripheral lamellar relaxation: a mechanism of induced corneal flattening in PTK and PRK? *Invest. Ophthalmol. Vis. Sci.,* 1995, 36, S708.

[75] Fernandez DC, Niazy AM, Kurtz RM, Djotyan GP, Juhasz T. Finite element analysis applied to corneal reshaping. *J. Biomed. Optics*., 2005, 10, 0640181-11.

[76] Djotyan GP, Kurtz RM, Fernandez DC, Juhasz T. An analytically solvable model for biomechanical response of the cornea to refractive surgery. Transactions of ASME, 2001, 123, 440-445.

[77] Bryant MR, McDonnel PJ. Constitutive laws for biomechanical modeling of refractive surgery. *J. Biomech. Eng.*, 1996, 118, 473-481.

[78] Alastrué V, Calvo B, Peña E, Doblaré M. Biomechanical Modeling of refractive corneal surgery. Transactions of ASME 2006, 128, 150-160.

[79] Katsube N, Wang R, Okuma E, Roberts C. Biomechanical response of the cornea to phototherapeutic keratectomy when treated as a fluid-filled porous material. *J. Refract. Surg.*, 2002, 18, S593-S597.

[80] Serrao S, Lombardo G, Lombardo M. Differences in nasal and temporal responses of the cornea after photorefractive keratectomy. *J. Cataract Refract. Surg.*, 2005; 31, 30-38.

[81] Olson R, Mamalis N, Haugen B. A light adjustable lens with injectable optics. *Curr. Opin. Ophthalmol.,* 2006, 17, 72-79.

[82] Sabesan R, Jeong TM, Carvalho L, Cox IG, Williams DR, Yoon G. Vision improvement by correcting higher-order aberrations with customized soft contact lenses in keratoconic eyes. *Opt. Lett.*, 2007, 32, 1000-1002.

[83] Li G, Mathine DL, Valley P, Ayras P, Haddock JN, Gridhar MS, Williby G, Schwiegerling J, Meredith GR, Kippelen B, Honkanen S, Peyghambarian N. Switchable electro-optic diffractive lens with high efficiency for ophthalmic applications. *PNAS*, 2006, 103, 6100-6104.

[84] Ye M, Wang B, Sato S. Liquid-crystal lens with a focal length that is variable in a wide range. *Appl. Opt*., 2004, 43, 6407-6412.

[85] Simonov AN, Vdovin G, Loktev M. Liquid-crystal intraocular adaptive lens with wireless control. *Opt. Expr.,* 2007, 15, 7468- 7478.

# Short Communications

In: Laser Keratectomy: Approaches, Complications... ISBN 978-1-60456-863-9
Author: Luis W. Schröder and Felix J. Walter 

*Short Communication A*

# Is PRK Induced Negative Spherical Aberration a Possible Way of Presbyopia Correction?

***A. Fea* [1]*, E. Amasio*[2]*, E. Bartoli* [1,2] *and F.M. Grignolo* [1]**
[1] Dipartimento di Fisiopatologia Clinica- Clinica Oculistica – Universita' di Torino
[2] LAS. E. R Srl Torino, Italy

## Introduction

Although the excimer laser correction of myopic and hyperopic defects has gained high levels of predictability and stability, the surface correction of presbyopia is still a matter of debate. It is well known that during accommodation in the pre-presbyopic age there is a change from slightly negative or neutral to a positive spherical aberration. Furthermore, when a hyperopic correction in a presbyopic patient is performed), it is commonly seen a better performance in near vision and a positive spherical aberration is usually induced. This observations lead to the idea that there might be a connection between spherical aberration (z4,0) and near vision. We present the 2 year's follow-up visual results of the treatment of myopic and hyperopic patients with the Zeiss Mel 70 Mel 80 excimer laser inducing a positive spherical aberration in 53 patients (Bartoli-Zeiss method).

## Materials and Methods

94 eyes (50 myopic eyes, 17 patients; 44 hyperopic eyes, 16 patients) were treated between 2004 and 2005 with the Mel 70 or Mel 80 excimer laser (Zeiss). The mean age of the myopic group (12 males, 15 females) was 45,1 ± 3,8 years (range: 40-57), in the hyperopic group ( 18 males, 8 females) mean age was 54.1 ± 7.1 years (range: 38-65). Near (Jaeger) and far visual acuity (ETDRS), contrast sensitivity (MAV, Sifi, Italy) were measured before surgery and at 1,2,3,6, 12 and 24 months.

Results: The mean near addiction was 1.48 ± 0.48 Diopters for the myopes and 2.29 ± 0.45 D for the hyperopes corresponding to a Z (4,0) of 0.128 μ . No net change in best spectacle corrected visual acuity was seen after the treatment (Myopes before: 0,90 ± 0,16, after: 0,93 ± 0,08; hyperopes: before: 0,94 ± 0,12, after: 0,96±0,13). In the Myopic group 10% of patients gained 2 or more line of BSCVA; in the hyperopic group, 9% gained 2 lines and 3% lost 2 lines of BSCVA. Monocular uncorrected near vision was 1.18 ± 0.41 J for myopes and 1.34 ± 0.47 J for hyperopes.

Conclusions: A slight improvement in near visual acuity was obtained by inducing a positive spherical aberration during a standard surface excimer laser treatment, without significant loss of far BSCVA. No significant complications were observed although x patients had the occurrence of haze and y complained of night vision problems (glare). The induction of a positive spherical aberration corresponds to a -0.185 ± 0.31 μ in hyperopes and to a 0.93 ± 0.38 μ in myopes. Thus in hyperopes a hypercorrection and in myopes a hypocorrection are needed in order to obtain emmetropia for far. The conceptual implication of this treatment are thoroughly discussed.

In: Laser Keratectomy: Approaches, Complications... ISBN 978-1-60456-863-9
Author: Luis W. Schröder and Felix J. Walter


*Short Communication B*

# Excimer Laser Surgery: A Watchful Eye for the Future

***Marco Lombardo*[*1,2], Maria Penelope De Santo [2], Giuseppe Lombardo [1,2], Riccardo Barberi [2], Lucia Ziccardi [3], and Sebastiano Serrao [3]***

[1] Vision Engineering, Reggio Calabria and Rome, Italy
[2]INFM-CNR LiCryL Laboratory, Physics Department, University of Calabria, Arcavacata di Rende (CS), Italy
[3]Serraolaser, Rome, Italy

## Abstract

Excimer laser corneal surgery allows the precise removal of tissue and it is nowadays used worldwide for the correction of the eye's optical aberrations. During the last years, novel methods and techniques have been developed in order to improve the accuracy of surface ablation surgery. On the other hand, even in an era of high-precision treatment algorithms, discrepancies between the intended and realized visual outcomes are sometimes manifest. The biophysical responses of the cornea undermine the predictability and stability of refractive surgery and contribute to these discrepancies.

Numerous factors depending on the ablation parameters may vary the remodeling of the ablated corneal surface leading to abnormal wound healing. A smooth postoperative stromal surface is required to achieve a high-quality visual outcome. In this work, we provide nanometer-resolved images of either native or photoablated corneas to demonstrate the opportunity in which Atomic Force Microscopy (AFM) may be valuable to understand the laser-tissue interaction and characterize the three-dimensional ultra-structural changes of the corneal stroma induced by excimer laser surgery.

The stromal surface of eight porcine corneas, both natural and photoablated, was imaged with AFM operating in balanced salt solution and contact mode. The AFM images of the intact corneal stroma, exposed after chemical removal of the epithelium,

* Address correspondence to: Dr. Marco Lombardo, MD, PhD, via Adda, 7 – 00198, Rome – ITALY, Phone and Fax: +39 06 88 40 971, E-mail: mlombardo@visioeng.it

showed a smooth surface with pores of varying diameter and dimension consisting in the Bowman's layer. Following ablation, the stromal surface showed undulations and micro-granular structures. These structures are considered to be either collapsed collagen fibrils and debris, directly due to the effects of laser beam impact onto the stromal surface. Topographical data, calculated using the section analysis module of the AFM software, showed an increased roughness of the post-ablated stromal surface compared to its native state, with a mean *root mean square roughness* value of 215 ± 49 nanometer (nm) and 144 ± 41 nm respectively. Nevertheless, the quantitative analysis proved that the laser cut of commercial excimer laser systems is very precise in removing even infinitesimally small amounts of tissue.

## Introduction

Excimer laser corneal surgery has become one of the most widely employed surgical techniques in Ophthalmology. Photorefractive surgery, by means of a 193 nm wavelength laser beam generated by a gas mixture of Argon and Fluorine (ArF), remodels the profile of the cornea and minimizes the refractive defects of the eye. The laser by its impact on the corneal plane breaks, through a photochemical interaction termed *photoablation*, the covalent organic bonds of the stromal collagen fibers, hence removing the corneal tissue with extreme precision. Different techniques for reshaping the corneal profile are used worldwide, as photorefractive keratectomy (PRK), laser epithelial keratomileusis (LASEK), laser assisted in situ keratomileusis (LASIK) [1] and epi-LASIK [2].

During the last decade, photorefractive surgery has undergone rapid technological development. The individualized correction of the eye optical aberrations will be the next golden standard of refractive surgery allowing all the patients treated to achieve their optimal individual visual perception. Customized ablation, linking the measurement of ocular wavefront aberrations and treatment, aims to eliminate low-order ocular aberrations, i.e., the sphero-cylindrical errors, whilst minimizing high-order aberrations [3,4,5].

On the other hand, the ultimate visual outcome of excimer laser refractive surgery depends on the biophysical response of the corneal tissue, that definitely represents the limiting factor for this type of surgery [6]. The biomechanical changes of the cornea induced by ablation and the epithelial and stromal healing are the two biophysical issues involved in the variability of the individual response to laser surgery. It is well known that the final corneal profile, and thus the corneal optical quality, after surgical reshaping of the cornea is a function of the biomechanical response of the tissue to a change in its structure. Predicting the biomechanical response is one of the major challenges of customized, aberration-reducing ablative procedures [7]. In addition, it is widely held that a smooth post-ablation surface is mandatory if refractive surgery is to be considered effective: an abnormal epithelial-stromal reaction of the ablated cornea is the consequence of an imperfectly polished ablated surface [8]. A smooth stromal surface is at the basis of an improved refractive result and it is associated with an increased predictability and stability of the final visual outcome [9]. Also, the more the postoperative corneal surface micrometric irregularities, the greater will the amount of induced high-order aberrations be [10], thus resulting in a decrease of visual performance.

The goal of research in this setting is to improve outcomes and reduce complications by discerning details of the biophysical pathways, identifying measurable predictors of individual responses and developing appropriate models for controlling or compensating for these factors.

A complete and correct knowledge of the ultra-structure of the photoablated corneal surface will allow ophthalmic surgeons and laser manufacturers to better test the ablation parameters and consequently improve the effectiveness of future customized refractive surgery [11,12].

The aim of the present study is to examine the effect of excimer laser treatment on porcine corneas using Atomic Force Microscopy (AFM) [13] and display the three dimensional characteristics of the ablated surface with respect to the natural one.

## Materials and Methods

Eight enucleated porcine fresh eye globes were used for this study, half of which underwent photorefractive keratectomy (PRK). Ablations of specimens were performed using the Technolas Keracor 217C excimer laser (Bausch and Lomb, Dornach, Germany). A laser technique was employed to excise the corneal epithelium [14] and then an ablation zone of 4.00 mm in diameter with a maximum depth of 80 micron (μm) was performed [15,16,17,18]. The non ablated porcine eyes were incubated in the presence of EDTA (2.5 mM) for 2 hours and the epithelium was then gently removed in order to expose the native anterior stromal surface.

The corneal surface was washed with a jet of saline solution prior to fixation and then all the corneal specimens, both natural as well as photoablated, were immediately fixed in situ by topical application and anterior chamber injection of a 2.5% glutaraldehyde solution [19]. All the eyes were conserved at a temperature of 4°C for 24 hours in the glutaraldehyde solution. Previous works [20,21] stated that the fixation procedure we used does not alter the surface of specimens compared to fresh unprepared ones and also facilitates the acquisition of high-resolution images. Therefore, the corneas were excised using a Hessburg-Barron trephine in order to obtain corneal specimens with a diameter of 8.00 mm. This procedure minimizes any possible alteration in the structure of the specimens themselves [22]. All the specimens were placed on the microscope sample holder and glued with cyanoacrylate glue with the endothelial side facing downwards. Maximum attention was paid during these maneuvers not to damage the corneal surface.

As group of control, we analyzed with AFM four human hairs either intact or after photoablation of exposed regions using a custom aluminum mask. A maximum ablation depth of 60 μm has been performed. The hairs were glued at the edges, paying maximum care in order not to deform their biological structure, on the sample holder.

Atomic Force Microscopy allows a three-dimensional (3-D) topographic reconstruction of the investigated sample on a nanometric scale (Figure 1). A commercially available Atomic Force Microscope (Autoprobe CP, Veeco, Sunnyvale, CA) was operated in balanced salt solution (BSS) in contact operating mode [15,16,18], using a V-shaped silicon nitride gold coated cantilever with a spring constant of 0.01 N/m (Veeco Metrology Group,

Sunnyvale, CA). The vertical resolution of the instrument is in the order of 0.1 nm. All the reported images were acquired with a 256 x 256 points resolution with scan rates of 1 to 5 Hz per line.

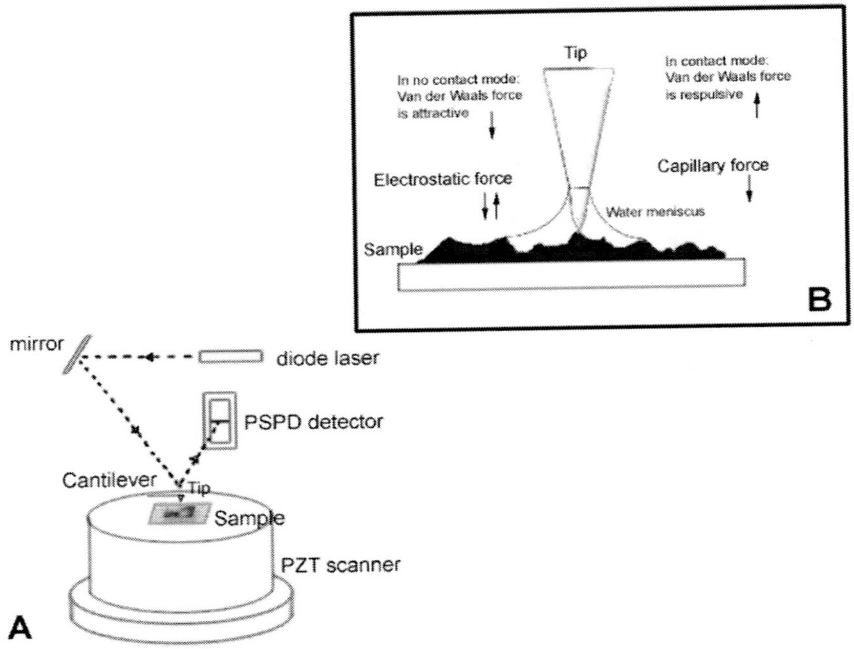


Figure 1. A) In AFM, the sample is scanned by a tip which is mounted on a flexible cantilever. While scanning, the forces between the tip and the sample cause bending of the cantilever. The deflection is monitored through an optical system, consisting of a laser diode and a position sensitive photo-detector (PSPD). The laser beam hits the reflective back of the cantilever and is reflected in the two-segmented photodiode. The PSPD itself permits a light displacement resolution less than one nm. The topography of the sample is obtained by plotting the deflections of the cantilever as a function of its position on the sample. With an appropriate feedback system, the deflection of the cantilever can be kept constant while the tip scans the specimen. During measurement, the specimen is driven by a piezoelectric scanner under the tip.

B) Several forces typically contribute to the deflection of the cantilever. The force most commonly associated with atomic force microscopy is an interatomic force called the Van der Waals force, the magnitude of which is in the range of nanoNewton (nN). Electrostatic forces and capillary forces between the tip and the sample are also involved.

An AFM may operate in contact or in no-contact mode. When the microscope operates in contact mode the tip scans the sample in close contact (a few Ångstroms) with the surface. The force on the tip is repulsive and has a magnitude of $10^{-7}$-$10^{-6}$ Newton (N). In no-contact mode, the tip is held at about one hundred Ångstroms from the surfaces. Hence, the forces between the tip and the sample are weaker than the ones in contact mode and approximate $10^{-12}$ N.

A single area on the cornea was imaged twice obtaining the same results, in order to ensure that the force exerted was not sufficient to damage the sample surface causing artifacts. Multiple imaging techniques were used to minimize the possibility that artifacts introduced by fixation could be misinterpreted as surface features. High-quality images were obtained within a wide range of image magnification. On the other hand, the area scanned was limited to a maximum of 50 $\mu m^2$ owing to the gross curvature of the cornea.

**Table 1. Average (± SD) quantitative analysis of the surface roughness of eight porcine corneas by means of RMS roughness value within a 10 $\mu m^2$ reference surface area**

| | RMS *roughness* (nanometer, M ± SD)* |
|---|---|
| Native Stroma (exposed Bowman's layer; 4 samples) | 144 ± 41 nm |
| Ablated stroma (4 samples) | 215 ± 49 nm |

* Student's *t*-test: $P<.05$.

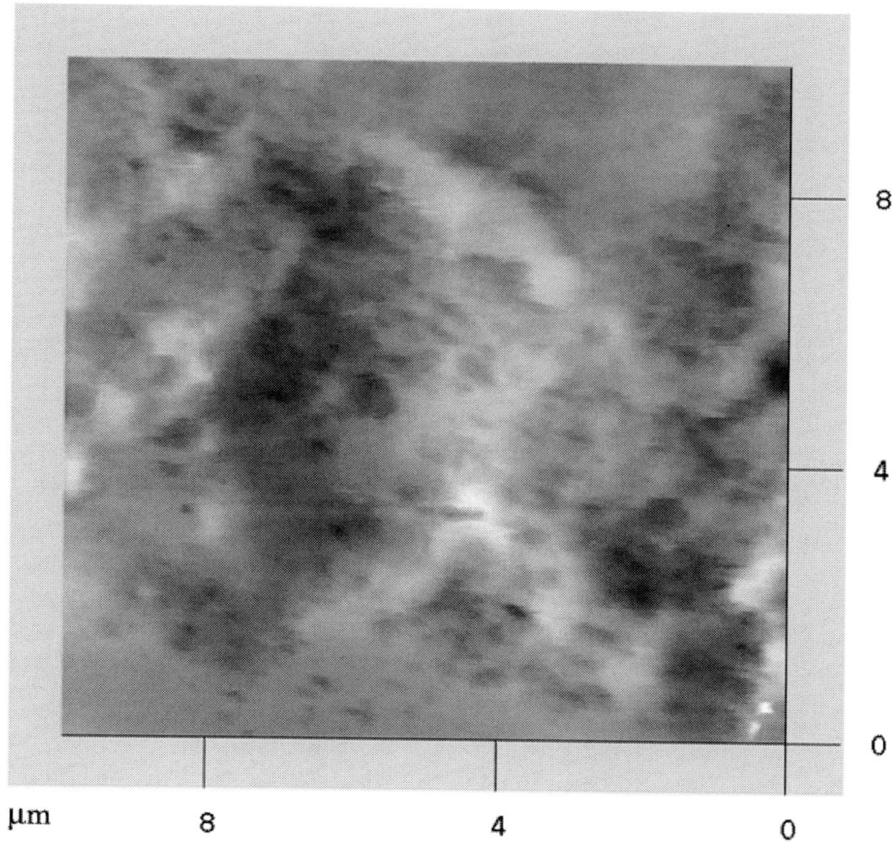


Figure 2. AFM image of the Bowman's layer. The Bowman's layer shows a complex topography of pores of varying sizes. Note the felt-like architecture of the surface. This complex topography provides an interface for cell-substratum interaction, it may also allow for the diffusion of components or for the passage of the nerves into the overlying epithelial layers. In the map, black corresponds to low features and white to high features (image size: 10 x 10 μm).

A set of images were taken from different areas close to the center of the corneal surface of the single specimen, both for the original and photoablated corneas.

All the images used for roughness measurement were processed using the specific AFM software. Processing included only flattening ($2^{nd}$ order) to remove the background slope due to the nonlinearities of the piezoelectric AFM scanner. Moreover, profile measurements and quantitative characterization of the surface roughness were achieved again using the AFM software. This allows measurements of linear distance and selection of one or more sections of the image for region analysis. Surface roughness measurements were made by calculating the root mean square value of the roughness within the given area (RMS roughness), i.e., the standard deviation of the height data. The surface roughness of the corneal stroma was evaluated by calculating the RMS roughness on reference surface areas of 10 $\mu m^2$. The same procedure was followed for the analysis of hairs. The Student's paired *t*-test was used to compare the differences in *RMS roughness* values between native and photoablated surfaces. A *P* value less than 0.05 was considered statistically significant.

## Results

Observation of the untreated corneas revealed a porous surface with pores of different depth and diameter, consisting in the Bowman's layer (Figure 2). The quantitative analysis of the Bowman's layer revealed a very smooth surface, as summarized in table 1.

The laser light output was the same we are used to set in clinical procedures, with fluence 120 $mJ/cm^2$, ablation rate 0.25 μm per pulse and the repetition rate 50 Hz. We selected the depth of ablation (80 μm and 60 μm for corneal specimens and hairs respectively) on the basis of the literature which proved that deeper treatments give rise to high surface irregularities [13,14,15,16].

Following ablation, the corneal surface was relatively rough showing undulations and micro-granular structures (Figure 3). Collagen fibrils arrangement areas were randomly displayed between these features that could represent the *pseudo-membrane* reported in scanning electron microscopy (SEM) studies [23]. The topographical analysis of the photoablated corneal specimens (the roughness measurements were performed on 50 areas of 10 $\mu m^2$ for statistical purpose) showed a significant increase ($P<.05$) in the surface roughness values in compare with the non ablated specimens.

AFM showed the hair cuticle consisting of scales of keratin lamellae. AFM images also clearly showed the longitudinal striations on the surface of the original hair's cuticle (Figure 4). The hair surface was very smooth along the non-ablated zones [24]. On the other hand, the ablated zones showed a diffuse granular topography at various magnification scales, probably due to the thermal effect generated by the ArF irradiation (Figure 5). The analysis has been performed on 50 areas of 10 $\mu m^2$. Results of the topographical analysis are summarized in Table 2. No significant differences ($P>.05$) between native and photoablated hairs' regions have been measured.

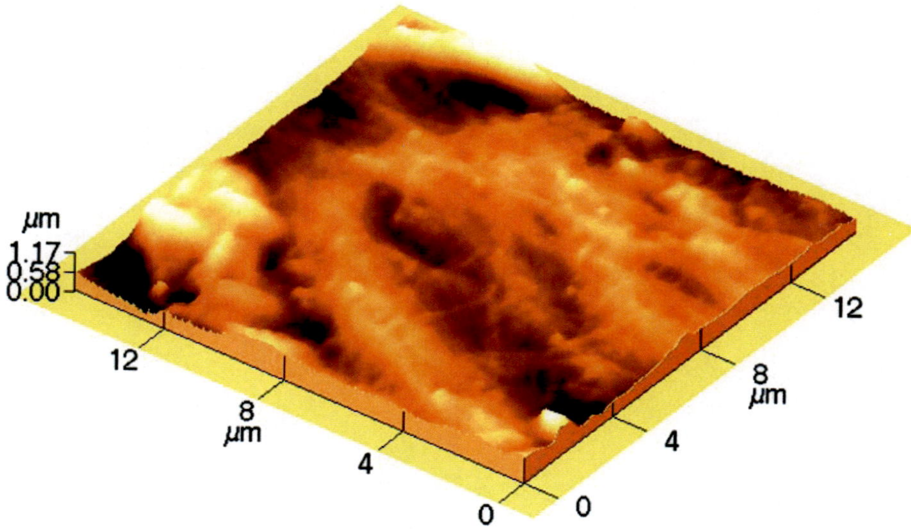


Figure 3. Three-dimensional view produced by AFM from the corneal stromal surface after standard eight diopters (maximum depth of ablation: 80 µm) photorefractive keratectomy. The image clearly shows undulations and granules as a result of the photoablative effect of the excimer laser at nano scale observation. Collagen fibrils are displayed between these features. Image size: 15 x 15 µm.

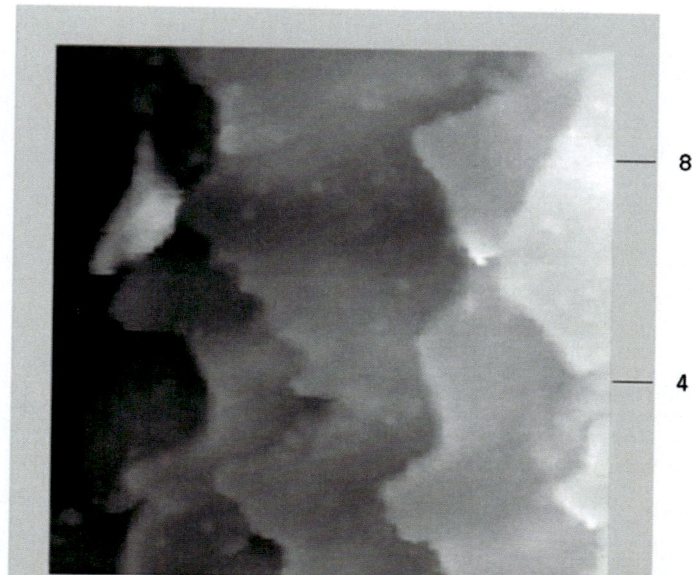


Figure 4. A three-dimensional AFM image of a natural human hair is shown. The surface appears to be very smooth. The steps correspond to the cuticular edges. Image size: 10 x 10 µm.

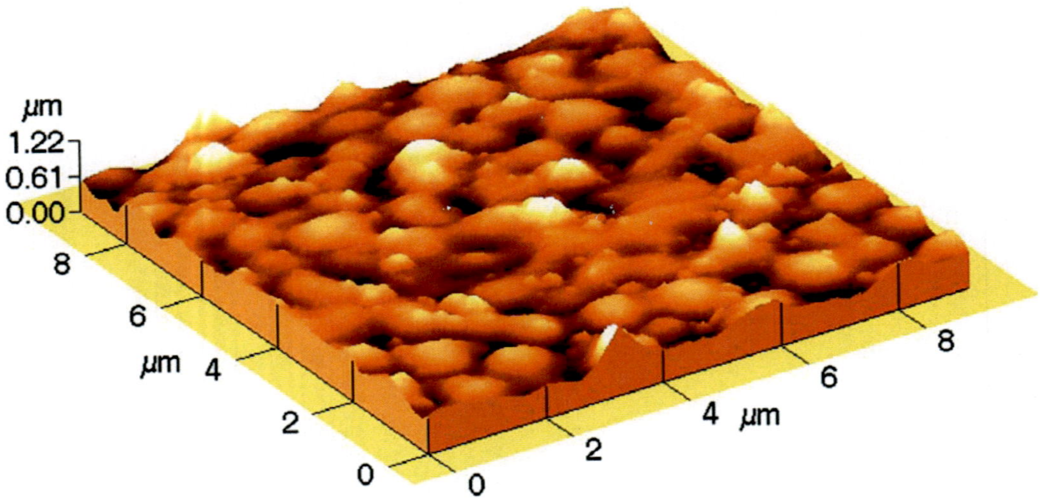


Figure 5. AFM three-dimensional image of a human hair after 60 μm depth photoablation. The sample surface shows a diffuse granular structure. These features may be directly dependent on the radiant and thermal effects of excimer laser onto the tissue. Image size: 10 μm x 10 μm.

**TABLE 2. Average (± SD) quantitative analysis of the surface roughness of four human hairs by means of RMS roughness value within a 10 μm² reference surface area**

| | RMS *roughness* (nanometer, M ± SD)† |
|---|---|
| Non ablated hair (2 samples) | 68 ± 37 nm |
| Ablated hair (2 samples) | 82 ± 34 nm |

† Student's *t*-test: *P*>.05.

# Conclusion

During the last decade, photorefractive surgery has dramatically evolved with the simultaneous development of more accurate laser platforms and diagnostic instruments, such as corneal topographers or ocular wavefront sensors. The development of videokeratoscopes, capable of recording the corneal shape in detail, and aberrometers, that measure the eye's wave aberration, has revealed that although standard laser refractive surgery eliminates conventional refractive errors, high-order errors are typically induced [25].

A better understanding of the biophysical properties of the corneal tissue may allow the prediction and modulation of its response to laser ablation for more precise correction; for that reason, it is required a detailed analysis of either the biomechanical or epithelial/stromal postoperative remodeling of the cornea.

A smooth post-ablation surface is the principal issue to prevent an abnormal remodeling of the ablated tissue [26,27]. The more are the surface architectural irregular modifications induced by the ablation the more delayed will the wound healing be. This phenomenon leads to an irregular remodeling of both the epithelium and stroma and consequently to an increase in the amount of postoperative high-order aberrations. An uniform distribution intensity of the laser beam over the entire treatment zone is the first essential requirement to achieve a quite smooth ablated surface. Numerous factors depending on the ablation parameters may vary the remodeling of the ablated corneal surface: i.e., the homogeneity of the laser impulse, which must pass through a long optic route within the laser cavity and resist the variable conditions of humidity and temperature within the operating theatre before impacting onto the corneal plane [28]; the overlapping of the laser impulses until the complete removal of the predicted amount of corneal tissue has been achieved; the ejected molecular ablated debris deposited back onto the corneal surface and the adsorption of the UV excimer laser beam in the plume as a consequence of the corneal ablation [28]; the not negligible thermal effect, associated with laser photoablation, due to temperature higher than 40°C, at which the collagen fibers of the corneal stroma are denatured [29]; the inclination of the ocular plane [11] and the saccadic movements of the eye.

Since the publication of the first article on photorefractive surgery by S. Trokel et al. in 1983 [30], numerous experimental and clinical studies documenting the efficacy and safety of excimer laser surgery and the ultramicroscopic characteristics of the corneal surface on which excimer laser ablation had been performed, have been published [10,12,14,16,18,23]. However, a systematic approach to the physical phenomena and especially to the laser-tissue interaction is lacking in the literature. Many authors involved in the investigation of the excimer laser-related phenomena have performed experimental studies ablating different biological tissues [12,15,16,30]; this, in order to compare and validate the dependence of the changes occurring on the ablated corneas to the ablation parameters.

In this work, we investigated the smoothness and the sub-microscopic topographic characteristics of corneal specimens using a nano-resolved imaging technique, namely Atomic Force Microscopy.

AFM techniques allow the examination of biological samples with minimal preparation and hence with a low risk of altering the surface details [31,32]. Moreover, a nanometer resolved imaging of the three dimensional topography of ablated surfaces may yield valuable information about the influence of laser beams on tissues. Human hairs were also analyzed before and after photoablation; this in order to compare the impact of excimer laser on different soft biological tissues. The choice to examine the hair has been based on its physical properties, similar to those of the corneal tissue, constituted by regular overlapping lamellae of protein macromolecules and a smooth surface profile. Such a surface allowed us to demonstrate the accuracy of the laser beam reshaping and also to measure, on a nanometric scale, the irregularities induced by photoablation.

The proper method of imaging the corneal surface was determined by reviewing the literature [15,16,18,20] and based on results of our previous experiments [12, 33]: the AFM was operated in contact mode in BSS, using triangular cantilevers with a very low elastic constant.

AFM imaging of the untreated stromal surface revealed a smooth layer, with micro depressions of varying depth and dimensions. These features are considered to be the pores of the Bowman's layer which have been observed at SEM [34]. To date, only one work reporting similar observations made at AFM has been published in the literature [15]. The significance of the pores could be twofold: they could constitute the site through which nerve fibers pass [35], or else a sort of anchoring structure which helps epithelial cells to migrate [36]. The Bowman's layer is the natural plane on which the epithelial cells migrate and stratify, hence it has been hypothesized that a smooth and regular surface may favor the natural healing process of the corneal epithelium [36].

Images acquired following photoablation revealed micro irregularities on the exposed stroma. The changes occurring in the topography of the corneal plane after photoablation may be directly due to the effects of the laser beam impact onto the surface: the *pseudo-membrane* is considered to be a thin superficial zone of damage specific to 193-nm ArF laser irradiations that results in coagulation of the collagen fibrils [29,37,38]. The granular structures are considered to be either collapsed collagen fibrils and debris [12,16,17]. Additionally, authors have demonstrated that fragments of materials, induced by boiling water solutions of the tissue during ablation, are ejected from the ablated surface into the gaseous state, meaning that a thermal loading is produced during the photorefractive procedure [39]. Undulations and granules observed at nano-scale images are not to be related to the irregular overlapping of the laser impulses that becomes more important at the lower magnification scale imaging obtained with wave optics microscopic techniques.

The photoablated hair showed a nano-surface topography similar to that noticed in the corneal specimens, with undulations and granules, likely due to a similar thermal effect on either keratin or collagen macromolecules. Differences in the granular appearance and induced surface roughness between the ablated surface of the hairs and that of the corneas may be related to the lesser water content [40] and the different mechanical properties of keratinous tissues compared to collagenous tissues.

In conclusion, in this work, we reported nanometric changes in the three dimensional topographic architecture of the ablated stroma and an increased surface roughness in all the ablated specimens. Nevertheless, the quantitative analysis confirmed the precision of commercial excimer laser devices in removing infinitesimally small amounts of tissue.

Research efforts are ongoing to understand the laser-corneal tissue interaction and also predict and modulate the epithelial and stromal healing in order to optimize refractive and visual outcomes of laser refractive surgery. Novel methods and techniques are regularly developed in order to improve the accuracy of surface ablation surgery, as, for example, advanced surface ablation (ASA) procedures [9,12, 41].

# References

[1] Munnerlyn CR, Koons SJ, Marshall J. Photorefractive keratectomy: a technique for laser refractive surgery. *J Cataract Refract Surg*, 1988,14, 46-52.

[2] Pallikaris IG, Katsanevaki V.J., Kalyvianaki MI, Naoumidi II. Advances in subepithelial excimer refractive surgery techniques: Epi-LASIK. *Curr Opin Ophthalmol*, 2003, 14, 207-212.

[3] Thibos LN. The prospects for perfect vision. *J Refract Surg*, 2000, 16, S540-S546.

[4] Applegate RA. Limits to vision: can we do better than nature? *J Refract Surg*, 2000,16, S547-S551.

[5] Kanjani N, Jacob S, Agarwal A, Agarwal A, Agarwal S, Agarwal T, Doshi A, Doshi S. Wavefront- and topography-guided ablation in myopic eyes using Zyoptix. *J Cataract Refract Surg*, 2004, 30, 398-402.

[6] Roberts C. The cornea is not a piece of plastic. *J Refract Surg*, 2000,16, 407-409.

[7] Roberts C. Biomechanics of the cornea and wavefront-guided laser refractive surgery. *J Refract Surg*, 2002, 18, S589-S592.

[8] Netto MV, Mohan RR, Ambrosio R, Hutcheon AEK, Zieske JD,. Wilson SE. Wound Healing in the Cornea. A Review of Refractive Surgery Complications and New Prospects for Therapy. *Cornea*, 2005, 24, 509–522.

[9] Serrao S, Lombardo M. One-year results of photorefractive keratectomy with and without surface smoothing using the Technolas 217C Laser. *J Refract Surg*, 2004, 20, 444-449.

[10] Lombardo M, Serrao S. Smoothing of the ablated porcine corneas using the Technolas Keracor 217C and Nidek EC-5000 excimer lasers. *J Refract Surg*, 2004, 20, 450-453.

[11] Ginis HS, Katsanevaki VJ, Pallikaris IG. Influence of ablation parameters on refractive changes after phototerapeutic keratectomy. *J Refract Surg*, 2003, 19, 443-447.

[12] Lombardo M, De Santo MP, Lombardo G, Barberi R, Serrao S. Roughness of excimer laser ablated corneas with and without smoothing with atomic force microscopy. *J Refract Surg*, 2005, 21, 469-475.

[13] Binning G, Quate C, Gerber C. Atomic force microscope. *Phys Rev Lett*, 1986, 56, 930-939.

[14] Weiss RA, Liaw L-H L, Berns M, Amoils SP. Scanning electron microscopy comparison of corneal epithelial removal techniques before photorefractive keratectomy. *J Cataract Refract Surg*, 1999, 25, 1093-1096.

[15] Abrams GA, Goodman SL, Nealy PF, Franco M, Murphy CJ. Nanoscale topography of the basament membrane underlying the corneal epithelium of the rhesus macaque. *Cell Tissue Res*, 2000, 299, 39-46.

[16] Nogradi A, Hopp B, Revesz K, et al. Atomic force microscopic study of the human cornea following excimer laser keratectomy. *Exp Eye Res*, 2000, 70, 363-368.

[17] Taylor ST, Fields CR, Barker FM, et al. Effect of depth upon the smoothness of excimer laser corneal ablation. *Opt Vis Sci*, 1994, 71, 104-108.

[18] Lydataki S, Lesniewska E, Tsilimbaris MK, Panagopoulou S, Le Grimellec G., Pallikaris IG. Excimer laser ablated cornea observed by atomic force microscopy. *Single Mol*, 2002, 2-3, 141-147.

[19] Doughty MJ. On the evaluation of the corneal epithelial surface by scanning electron microscopy. *Optom Vis Sci*, 1990, 67, 735-756.

[20] Tsilimbaris MK, Lesniewska E, Lydataki S, Le Grimellec C, Goudonnet JP, Pallikaris IG. The use of atomic force microscopy for the observation of corneal epithelium surface. *Invest Ophthalmol Vis Sci*, 2000, 41, 680-686.

[21] Sinniah, K, Paauw, J, Ubels, J. Investigating live and fixed epithelial and fibroblast cells by atomic force microscopy. *Curr Eye Res*, 2002; 25, 61-68

[22] Damiano RE, Van Horn DL, Schultz RO. Trephination of donor corneal buttons: a scanning electron microscopic study. *Ann Ophthalmol*, 1978, 10, 479-485.

[23] Kerr-Muir MG, Trokel SL, Marshall J, Rothery S. Ultrastructural comparison of conventional surgical and argon fluoride excimer laser keratectomy. *Am J Ophthalmol*, 1987, 103, 448-453.

[24] Smith JR. A quantitative method for analysing AFM images of the outer surfaces of human hair, *J Microsc*, 1998, 191, 223-228.

[25] Williams D, Yoon GY, Porter J, Guirao A, Hofer H, Cox I. Visual benefit of correcting higher order aberrations of the eye. *J Refract Surg*, 2000, 16, S554-S559.

[26] Weber BA, Gan L, Fagerholm P. Wound healing response in the presence of stromal irregularities after excimer laser treatment. *Acta Ophthalmol Scand*, 2001, 79, 381-388.

[27] Møller-Pedersen T, Cavanagh HD, Petroll WM, Jester JV. Stromal wound healing explains refractive instability and haze development after photorefractive keratectomy. *Ophthalmology*, 2000, 107, 1235-1245.

[28] Van Horn SD, Hovanesian JA, Maloney RK. Effect of volatile compounds on excimer laser power delivery. *J Refract Surg*, 2002, 18, 524-528.

[29] Maldonado-Codina C, Morgan PB, Efron N. Thermal consequences of photorefractive keratectomy. *Cornea*, 2001, 20, 509-515.

[30] Trokel SL, Srinivasan R, Braren B. Excimer laser surgery of the cornea. *Am J Ophthalmol*, 1983, 96, 710-715.

[31] Braet F, Kalle WH, De Zanger RB, et al. Comparative atomic force and scanning electron microscopy: an investigation on fenestrated endothelial cells in vitro. *J Microsc*, 1996, 181, 10-17.

[32] Poletti G, Orsini F, Lenardi C, et al. A comparative study between AFM and SEM imaging on human scalp hair. *J Microsc*, 2003, 21, 249-255.

[33] Lombardo M, De Santo MP, Lombardo G, Barberi R, Serrao S. Atomic Force Microscopy analysis of normal and photoablated porcine corneas. *J Biomechanics*, 2006, 39, 2719-2724.

[34] Abrams GA, Bentley E, Nealey PF, Murphy CJ. Electron microscopy of the canine corneal basement membranes. *Cells Tissues Organs*, 2002, 170, 251-257.

[35] Hayashi, S, Osawa, T, Tohyama, K. Comparative observations on corneas, with special reference to Bowman's layer and Descemet's membrane in mammals and amphibians. *J Morphol*, 2002, 254, 247-258.

[36] Dalton BA, McFarland GA, Steele JG. Stimulation of epithelial tissue migration by certain porous topographies is independent of fluid flux. *J Biomed Mater Res*, 2001, 56, 83-92.

[37] Betney S, Morgan PB, Doyle SJ, Efron N. Corneal temperature changes during photorefractive keratectomy. *Cornea*, 1997, 16, 158-161.

[38] Puliafito CA, Steinert RF, Deutsch TF, Hillenkamp EJ, Dehm CM. Adler . Excimer laser ablation of the cornea and lens. *Ophthalmology*, 1985, 92, 741-748.

[39] Hahn DW, Ediger MN, Pettit GH. Dynamics of ablation plume particles generated during excimer laser corneal ablation. *Lasers Surg Med*, 1995, 16, 384-389.

[40] DeMali KA, Williams TR. Determination of the content of water in bovine corneas by differential scanning calorimetry and thermogravimetric analysis. *Ophthalmic Res*, 1994, 26, 105-109.

[41] Randleman JB, Loft ES, Banning CS, Lynn MJ, Stulting RD. Outcomes of wavefront-optimized surface ablation. *Ophthalmology*, 2007, 114, 983-988.

# Index

## A

## D



## E

## F



## G



## H

## I



## K

## N



## O



## P

## Q



## R

## S

## W